Upper Facial Rejuvenation

Editor

FAISAL A. QUERESHY

ATLAS OF THE ORAL AND MAXILLOFACIAL SURGERY CLINICS OF NORTH AMERICA

www.oralmaxsurgeryatlas.theclinics.com

Consulting Editor
RICHARD H. HAUG

September 2016 • Volume 24 • Number 2

ELSEVIER

1600 John F. Kennedy Boulevard • Suite 1800 • Philadelphia, Pennsylvania, 19103-2899
http://www.oralmaxsurgeryatlas.theclinics.com

ATLAS OF THE ORAL AND MAXILLOFACIAL SURGERY CLINICS OF NORTH AMERICA Volume 24, Number 2
September 2016 ISSN 1061-3315 ISBN-13: 978-0-323-46251-8

Editor: John Vassallo; j.vassallo@elsevier.com
Developmental Editor: Colleen Viola

Reprints. For copies of 100 or more of articles in this publication, please contact the Commercial Reprints Department, Elsevier Inc., 360 Park Avenue South, New York, NY 10010-1710. Tel.: 212-633-3874; Fax: 212-633-3820; E-mail: reprints@elsevier.com.

Atlas of the Oral and Maxillofacial Surgery Clinics of North America (ISSN 1061-3315) is published biannually by Elsevier, 360 Park Avenue South, New York, NY 10010-1710. Months of issue are March and September. Periodicals postage paid at New York, NY and additional mailing offices. Subscription prices are $455.00 for international individual, $370.00 for US individual and Canadian individual; $220.00 for international student and Canadian student, $100.00 for US student; $489.00 for international institution, $515.00 for Canadian institution, $398.00 for US institution. Foreign air speed delivery is included in all *Clinics* subscription prices. All prices are subject to change without notice. POSTMASTER: Send address changes to *Atlas of the Oral and Maxillofacial Surgery Clinics of North America*, Health Sciences Division, Subscription Customer Service, 3251 Riverport Lane, Maryland Heights, MO 63043. Tel: 1-800-654-2452 (U.S. and Canada); 314-447-8871 (outside U.S. and Canada). Fax: 314-417-8029. E-mail: journalscustomerservice-usa@elsevier.com (for print support); journalsonline support-usa@elsevier.com (for online support).

Atlas of the Oral and Maxillofacial Surgery Clinics of North America is covered in *MEDLINE/PubMed (Index Medicus)*.

Printed in the United States of America.

Contributors

EDITOR

FAISAL A. QUERESHY, MD, DDS, FACS
Associate Professor; Residency Program Director;
Department of Oral and Maxillofacial Surgery/Facial Cosmetic
Surgery, Case Western Reserve University, Cleveland, Ohio;
Medical Director, Visage Surgical Institute, Medina, Ohio

AUTHORS

MEHMET ALI ALTAY, DDS, PhD
Department of Oral and Maxillofacial Surgery, Akdeniz
University, Antalya, Turkey

DALE A. BAUR, DDS
Department of Oral and Maxillofacial Surgery, Case Western
Reserve University, Cleveland, Ohio

MANIK BEDI, MD, DDS
Private Practice, Zephyrhills, Florida

ANGELO CUZALINA, MD, DDS
Fellowship Director, Private Practice, Tulsa Surgical Arts,
Tulsa, Oklahoma

HARDEEP DHALIWAL, MD, DMD
Private Practice, Redmond, Washington

HUSAM ELIAS, MD, DMD, FACS
Southern California Center for Surgical Arts, Sherman Oaks,
California

TIRBOD FATTAHI, MD, DDS, FACS
Chair, Department of Oral and Maxillofacial Surgery,
University of Florida, Jacksonville, Florida

JACOB HAIAVY, MD, DDS, FACS
Inland Cosmetic Surgery, Rancho Cucamonga, California;
Assistant Clinical Professor of Oral and Maxillofacial Surgery,
Loma Linda University, Loma Linda, California

DOUGLAS L. JOHNSON, DMD
Private Practice, Saint Augustine, Florida; Clinical Faculty
(Part Time), Department of Oral and Maxillofacial Surgery,
University of Florida, Jacksonville, Florida

GARY LINKOV, MD
Department of Otolaryngology – Head & Neck Surgery,
Temple University School of Medicine, Philadelphia,
Pennsylvania

SEAN PACK, DDS, MD
Department of Oral and Maxillofacial Surgery, Case Western
Reserve University, Cleveland, Ohio

FRANK PALETTA, MD, DMD, FACS
Private Practice, Warwick, Rhode Island; Clinical Assistant
Professor, Department of Surgery, Warren Alpert Medical
School of Brown University, Providence, Rhode Island;
Clinical Instructor, Division of Oral and Maxillofacial Surgery,
Department of Craniofacial Science, University of
Connecticut, Farmington, Connecticut

JON D. PERENACK, MD, DDS
Associate Clinical Professor, LSU Department of Oral and
Maxillofacial Surgery, New Orleans, Louisiana; Medical and
Surgical Director, Williamson Cosmetic Surgery Center,
Baton Rouge, Louisiana

CLEMENT QAQISH, MD, DDS
Private Practice, San Diego Surgical Arts, San Diego,
California

FAISAL A. QUERESHY, MD, DDS, FACS
Associate Professor; Residency Program Director;
Department of Oral and Maxillofacial Surgery/Facial Cosmetic
Surgery, Case Western Reserve University, Cleveland, Ohio;
Medical Director, Visage Surgical Institute, Medina, Ohio

CHRISTOPHER BLAKE SMITH, DMD, MD
Private Practice, Cosmetic and Facial Surgery of East
Alabama, Opelika, Alabama

PETER DANIEL WAITE, MPH, DDS, MD, FACS
Professor and Chairman, UAB Oral and Maxillofacial Surgery,
Birmingham, Alabama

MICHAEL J. WILL, MD, DDS, FACS
Medical Director, Will Surgical Arts, Ijamsville, Maryland

ALLAN E. WULC, MD, FACS
Department of Otolaryngology – Head & Neck Surgery,
Temple University School of Medicine; Clinical Associate
Professor, Department of Ophthalmology, Scheie Eye
Institute, University of Pennsylvania, Philadelphia,
Pennsylvania; Private Practice, W Cosmetic Surgery,
Plymouth Meeting, Pennsylvania

Contents

Preface: Rejuvenation of the Facial Upper Third   xi

Faisal A. Quereshy

Analysis and Diagnosis of Upper Facial Region   87

Hardeep Dhaliwal

    Introduction   87
    Patient evaluation   87
    Photo documentation   87
    Anatomic analysis   87
    Esthetic analysis by region   88
    Summary   93

Botulinum Toxin Use in the Upper Face   95

Clement Qaqish

    Introduction   95
    Preoperative planning and pretreatment assessment   95
    Procedural technique   98
    Complications   100
    After procedure care   101
    Outcomes   101
    Summary   102

Injectable Fillers in the Upper Face   105

Jacob Haiavy and Husam Elias

    ▶ Video content accompanies this article at http://www.oralmaxsurgeryatlas.theclinics.com.

    Introduction   105
    Surgical technique   105
    Glabellar folds   106
    Forehead lines   106
    Lateral canthal lines: (crow's feet)   106
    Periorbital, tear trough, nasojugal groove   107
    Temporal wasting hollowing   107
    Surgical technique of fat transfer   107
    Preoperative planning   107
    Preparation and patient positioning   107
    Surgical approach   108
    Surgical procedure   108
    Immediate postoperative care   110
    Potential complications   110
    Rehabilitation and recovery   112
    Clinical results in the literature   113
    Hyaloronic acid soft tissue fillers   114
    Sculptra-Poly-L-Lactic acid   115
    Autologous fat transfer   115
    Summary   115

Skin Resurfacing Procedures of the Upper Face

Douglas L. Johnson and Frank Paletta

▶ Video content accompanies this article at http://www.oralmaxsurgeryatlas.theclinics.com.

Introduction	117
Surgical technique	119
Rehabilitation and recovery	120
Summary	122

Upper Eyelid Blepharoplasty

Michael J. Will

Introduction	125
Anatomy of the periorbital region	125
Eyelid esthetics	127
Age-related changes of the periorbital region	127
Preoperative assessment	129
Selection of surgical procedure	129
Surgical planning and skin markings	129
Anesthesia considerations	129
Upper blepharoplasty procedure	130
Ancillary periorbital procedures	130
Postoperative care	131
Complications	131
Periorbital rejuvenation pearls	133

Lower Transcutaneous Blepharoplasty

Christopher Blake Smith and Peter Daniel Waite

Introduction	135
Preoperative planning	135
Preparation and patient markings	136
Patient positioning and surgical technique	137
Transconjuctival approach	137
Skin pinch technique	138
Skin-muscle flap approach	139
Incision and flap elevation	139
Orbital fat management	139
Orbicularis oculi muscle	141
Lower lid support	141
Skin excision	141
Complications	142
Bleeding	142
Lower eyelid malposition	143
Chemosis	144
Dry eyes	144
Postoperative care	144
Follow-up care	144
Summary	144

117

125

135

Transconjunctival Lower Blepharoplasty **147**

Sean Pack, Faisal A. Qureshy, Mehmet Ali Altay, and Dale A. Baur

Introduction 147
Anatomy 147
Pathophysiology of aging 148
Indications 149
Advantages and disadvantages 150
Technique 150
Complications 151
Discussion 151

Management of Lower Eyelid Laxity **153**

Gary Linkov and Allan E. Wulc

Introduction 153
Lateral canthal anatomy 153
Pathogenesis of eyelid laxity 154
Assessment 154
Procedures 156
Complications 158
Summary 159

Open Brow Lift Surgery for Facial Rejuvenation **161**

Tirbod Fattahi

Introduction 161
Patient selection 161
Surgical technique 162
Postoperative care 163
Summary 164

The Endoscopic Brow Lift **165**

Jon D. Perenack

Brow lift general considerations 165
Indications 165
Contraindications 165
Relative contraindications 165
Evaluation and diagnosis 165
Brow ptosis 165
Cosmetic botulinum toxin therapy 166
Skin 166
Clinical technique 166
Complications and controversies 172
Other considerations 173

Management of Complications Associated with Upper Facial Rejuvenation   **175**

Angelo Cuzalina and Manik Bedi

Introduction   175
Preoperative evaluation   175
Complications in browlift   176
Brow malposition   176
Nerve damage   177
Scars   178
Alopecia   178
Bleeding   179
Summary   179

ATLAS OF THE ORAL AND MAXILLOFACIAL SURGERY CLINICS OF NORTH AMERICA

FORTHCOMING ISSUES

March 2017

Management of Mandibular Condylar Fractures
Martin B. Steed, *Editor*

September 2017

Oral Manifestations of Systemic Diseases
Joel J. Napeñas, *Editor*

PREVIOUS ISSUES

March 2016

Techniques in Orthognathic Surgery
Steven M. Sullivan, *Editor*

September 2015

Adjuncts for Care of the Surgical Patient
Sidney L. Bourgeois Jr, *Editor*

March 2015

Diagnosis and Management of Neck Masses
David E. Webb, *Editor*

RELATED INTEREST

Oral and Maxillofacial Surgery Clinics of North America, May 2016, Volume 28, Issue 2
Management of the Cleft Patient
Kevin S. Smith, *Editor*
Available at: www.oralmaxsurgery.theclinics.com

THE CLINICS ARE NOW AVAILABLE ONLINE!

Access your subscription at:
www.theclinics.com

Preface

Rejuvenation of the Facial Upper Third

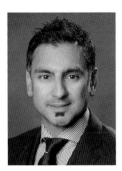

Faisal A. Quereshy, MD, DDS, FACS
Editor

I am honored to have been given the opportunity to share with you, our reader, this issue of *Atlas of the Oral and Maxillofacial Surgery Clinics of North America* on facial rejuvenation of the upper third. The upper face has always been simplified with treatment of isolated areas, such as eyelids only, but advances and innovations in facial cosmetic surgery medicine allow us to further define our techniques to offer patients a more comprehensive approach to rejuvenation.

We have been most fortunate to have experts from our field and allied colleagues support this issue with their expertise from years of clinical practice. Having contributions from the finest surgeons in facial cosmetic surgery, this issue presents information in a very clear, concise, and up-to-date manner that will allow readers of all backgrounds to benefit, either as review or to learn new techniques.

This issue will first embark on the nonsurgical therapies used to enhance upper facial regions with use of injectables and skin care regimens, followed by invasive treatment specific for brow and eyelid management. Pitfalls and complications are discussed. You will find this issue to be complete, with excellent illustrations supplemented with before and after photographs of treated individuals to punctuate the treatment results.

I would like to extend my gratitude to my esteemed colleagues for producing a high-quality issue that will surely become a mainstay for residents and future surgeons with a growing interest in facial cosmetic surgery. They have continued to push the scope of our specialty to the recognized level by our patients and peers. I am grateful for their continual guidance in teaching me to be a lifelong student of the profession. I hope you, the reader, will feel the same after reviewing our issue: Upper Facial Rejuvenation.

Faisal A. Quereshy, MD, DDS, FACS
Department of Oral and Maxillofacial Surgery
Case Western Reserve University
2124 Cornell Road
Room DOA 53A
Cleveland, OH 44106-4905, USA

E-mail address:
faq@case.edu

Atlas Oral Maxillofacial Surg Clin N Am 24 (2016) xi
1061-3315/16/$ - see front matter © 2016 Published by Elsevier Inc.
http://dx.doi.org/10.1016/j.cxom.2016.06.001

Analysis and Diagnosis of Upper Facial Region

Hardeep Dhaliwal, MD, DMD

KEYWORDS

- Upper facial • Evaluation • Brow • Eye • Blepharoplasty • Browlift • Esthetic • Diagnosis

KEY POINTS

- The upper facial region frames the eyes and thus has been one of major hallmarks of beauty for millennia.
- Cosmetic surgery in the region is one of most rewarding and sought after surgeries in the discipline.
- Evaluation, analysis, and diagnosis is of utmost importance in achieving optimal results; however, there is constant debate over the ideal method of analysis.
- The surgical management of this region is continually evolving in hopes of achieving the ideal result and ultimate patient and surgeon satisfaction.
- Preoperative planning is of utmost importance in minimizing postoperative complications.

Introduction

Facial esthetic analysis has a long and fundamental history in cosmetic surgery. There is continual debate on what is deemed to be esthetic and it continues to evolve. In addition, the views on facial esthetics can vary between ethnicities, cultures, geographies, and fashion trends. However, there are many key concepts that have not changed in centuries. Furthermore, the surgical intervention used to restore and improve facial esthetics is constantly evolving. The ideal assessment of beauty is a balance between the desires and wishes of a patient and his or her surgeon. The ultimate success is measured by a patient's satisfaction.

Patient evaluation

Patient evaluation is a very important aspect of the analysis of a potential cosmetic surgery patient. A thorough history and physical should be performed on all preoperative patients. In addition to the standard history and physical examination, a focused review of systems should be performed with focus of facials issues like vision changes, dry eyes, and so on. In addition, particular attention should be addressed to the use of over-the-counter supplements because they can alter healing and coagulation and thus have impact on surgical outcomes and incidence of complications.

The most critical aspect of the patient evaluation in the cosmetic surgery patient is obtaining a detailed chief complaint. Even if the surgical outcome of cosmetic surgery is outstanding, if it does not address the chief complaint, the final outcome is a failure. In some cases, the chief complaint may need to be modified by the patient, once the patient is counseled on the areas of interest. In addition, the patient's motivation for undergoing surgery is of critical significance; internal patient motivation will typically lead to highest rate of success. In cases where patient motivations are questionable or their expectations are not realistic, the ideal success may be referral of the patient to a different provider!

Photo documentation

Photo documentation is of critical importance in cosmetic surgery. It aids not only in the analysis and diagnosis of patients, but also serves to educate patients on the findings. Furthermore, not only can these photos help to educate the patient preoperatively, they can help to educate and inform patient postoperatively, particularly when patients are dissatisfied with their results. It is beyond the scope of this paper to discuss photo documentation in detail. The keys for successful photo documentation are taking all photos for all patients in the same fashion and same angle. For the face, it is particularly important to take photos with and without a flash to help accentuate shadows and contour deformities[1] that one wishes to improve or correct surgically. If preoperative and postoperative photos are taken with a flash only, the before and after photos will not do justice to the true result achieved. This may become less of an issue as 3-dimensional photography becomes more common.

Anatomic analysis

Traditionally, when analyzing the face in the vertical dimension, it is divided equally into thirds (Fig. 1). When dividing the facial height into thirds vertically, the top third extends form the hairline to glabella, the middle third extends from the glabella to the subnasale, and the lower third extends from the subnasale to menton.

The author has nothing to disclose.

Private Practice, 16517 Northeast 43rd Court, Redmond, WA 98052, USA

E-mail address: northwestcosmetic@gmail.com

Atlas Oral Maxillofacial Surg Clin N Am 24 (2016) 87–93
http://dx.doi.org/10.1016/j.cxom.2016.05.002

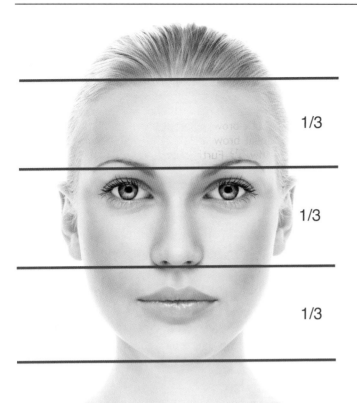

Fig. 1 Facial thirds. Ideal facial esthetics show equality between the vertical facial thirds. The face is divided into vertical thirds from the hairline to the glabella and glabella to subnasale and subnasale to menton. (© Valentina R. / Adobe Stock.)

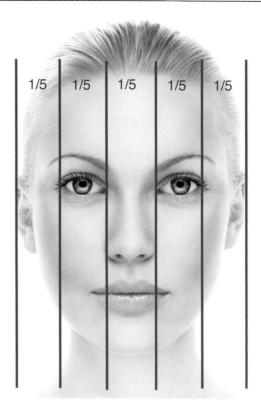

Fig. 2 Facial fifths. Ideal facial esthetics show equality between the horizontal facial fifths. The face is divided into horizontal fifths from pinnae of the ear to the lateral canthi and then to the medial canthi. (© Valentina R. / Adobe Stock.)

When analyzing the face in the horizontal dimension, it is divided equally in fifths (Fig. 2). The facial width is divided in fifths horizontally, the most lateral fifth extends from the pinna to the lateral canthus, the central fifth extends from medial canthus to medial, and the other fifth is the palpebral third, which extends form lateral canthus to the medial canthus. In addition, with analyzing the horizontal dimensions, it is considered balanced when the intercanthal distance is coincident with the alar bases.

It is considered esthetic when there is quantitative equality between these vertical thirds and horizontal fifths. Facial shapes arise from the interplay between the ratio of the facial thirds and fifths to each other. For example, longer faces will have longer facial thirds in comparison with the facial fifths.

In general, the face should have smooth flowing contours and these should be smooth and contiguous or complementary with adjacent facial areas. For example, the orbital rim continues a smooth flowing contour to the lateral aspect of the nose and the lower eyelid blends gently into the midface on a profile view.

Esthetic analysis by region

Forehead

The hairline can change overtime and thus its esthetic position does not always follow the "rule of thirds" for the face.[2–4] The other method used is the "curve of the head rule" and using the line drawn between the intersection of the horizontal line of the scalp with vertical line of the face. Thus, the hairline

rests somewhere on the curve joining these 2 planes.[5,6] In general, the hairline should be located 5 to 6 cm (5 cm in females and 6 cm in males) from the brow, in a patient with a nonreceded hairline.

Forehead convexity and inclination can play a significant role in the perceived forehead height.[7] A patient with a flat or protruding forehead will have an apparent shorter forehead compared with that of patient with a posteriorly sloping forehead.[7] In addition, recognizing the inclination of the forehead, its length, and the position of the hairline are important in preoperative planning of endoscopic procedures in the area. In general, ideal esthetics are seen with a forehead having a gently convex surface extending from the top of head to the brow (on a profile view).[7] The most anterior aspect of the forehead should be at the glabella just above the nasion. The nasofrontal angle should be 115° to 135°.

The prominence of the glabella and overlying soft tissues is quite important to forehead esthetics as well. The prominence is typically more profound in the male patient. Thus, many females with prominence in the area request the prominence to be addressed surgically. A lateral cephalometric radiograph can be useful in assessing bony contours in the area and for surgical planning should glabellar reduction be performed. Modification of the glabella and supraorbital ridge can play a very important role in the cosmetic surgery patient, particularly in facial feminization procedures.[8] If glabellar prominence is seen in combination with deep static glabeller rhytids and accentuated volume on dynamic contraction, the excess volume is likely from muscular hypertrophy. This muscular hypertrophy can be address through surgical excision or the use of neuromodulators.

Analysis of forehead static and dynamic rhytids are an important part of the facial analysis as well. Static rhytids develop over time in the forehead from contraction of the frontalis muscle from raising the brow. Rhytids over the glabella and nasal dorsum are from contraction of the corrugator supercilli muscle and procerus muscle. Dynamic rhytids can typically be addressed with neuromodulators or surgery; however, deeper static rhytids typically require operative intervention and skin resurfacing and possible volume augmentation.

Eyebrow

The eyebrows are defined by the hair growth in the area. In general, in the esthetic brow, the brow hairs have a general angle of orientation at the different aspects of the brow, at its most medial aspect the hair is oriented in superior direction and are then directed more laterally in the central brow and then continue to follow in parallel with the course of the brow.[7] With the degree of grooming that occurs in the area, the amount of hair remaining in the area is sometimes negligible, hence the increased amount of eyebrow tattooing seen in current times. These patients can sometimes be challenging to treat, particularly if the tattooing is placed at a higher level than where the native brow used to be.

The ideal brow architecture and position has been described by Westmore.[9,10] He described the brow (Fig. 3) as beginning medially along a vertical line running from nasal ala and medial canthus. The brown terminates laterally on the line running from the nasal ala to the lateral canthus. The peak of the arch of brow was described as being centered over a vertical line drawn from the lateral corneal limbus. This has been modified by many and there are number of other descriptions with slight variation, most notable being the peak of the arch being centered anywhere from the lateral limbis to the lateral canthus. Some studies have shown there to be no superior esthetic brow architecture. However, other studies have shown some brow architectures to be more esthetically pleasing, particularly when comparing different facial shapes.[11,12]

The ideal esthetic brow definition changes with age, sex and ethnicity. The ideal brow height also differs at different aspects of the brow.[9,13] Further complicating the matter are culture and current fashion trends, and the resulting grooming of the eyebrow can alter the natural brow position significantly.[9,13] Classically, the medial brow starts at or above the orbital rim and then arches superiorly moving laterally. The height of the arch is typically anywhere from the lateral corneal limbus to lateral canthus. However, in the male brow, there is typically less or an arch and it is positioned mostly over the orbital rim (Fig. 4).[14]

The top of the brow is typically 2.5 cm above the center of the pupil and 5 to 6 cm (5 cm in females and 6 cm in males; Fig. 5) below the hairline.[15] In the case of a receding hairline, these numbers can change; thus, other landmarks can be used to evaluate the hairline and brow. The brow has also been described as the lower edge being 15 to 16 mm above the upper eyelid crease.[16,17]

When assessing a patient for browptosis, it is imperative that any tonic contraction of the frontalis muscles is addressed. A simple method that may minimize muscle activity in the area is to ask the patient to relax their forehead and face and close their eyes, then manual pressure from the clinician's hands can aid in massaging and relaxing the brows.[18] The patient is then asked to slowly open the eyes and instructed not to move any surrounding muscles. During this short period of time the brows can be assessed in their static state with minimal muscle influences; however, the patient will typically quickly again activate the brow muscles. Thus, this maneuver may need to be repeated multiple times until a thorough evaluation of the brow is accomplished. Complicating things further is that many patients have asymmetrical heights of the brow. On certain patients, this brow asymmetry occurs concomitantly with the existence of orbital dystopia (Fig. 6). These findings should be discussed with a the patient before surgery, to ensure they understand the goals of surgery.

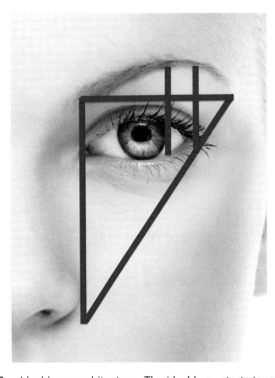

Fig. 3 Ideal brow architecture. The ideal brow starts tangential to the ala—medial canthus line and terminated tangential to the ala—lateral canthus line, with the peak of the brow occurring anywhere between the lateral corneal limbus to lateral canthus. (© Valentina R. / Adobe Stock.)

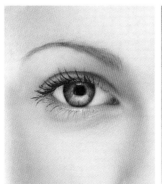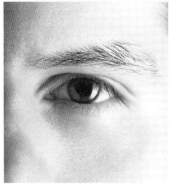

Fig. 4 Male versus female brow: Classically, the medial brow starts at or above the orbital rim and then arches superiorly moving laterally. The height of the arch is typically anywhere from the lateral corneal limbus to lateral canthus. However, in the male brow, there is typically less of an arch and it is positioned mostly over the orbital rim. (Left: © shefkate / Adobe Stock; Right: © eyeQ / Adobe Stock.)

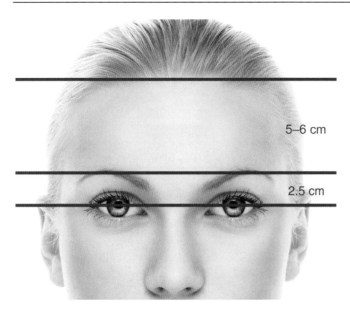

Fig. 5 Eyebrow heights. The top of the brow is typically 2.5 cm above the center of the pupil and 5 to 6 cm (5 cm in females and 6 cm in males) below the hairline. (© Valentina R. / Adobe Stock.)

Eyes

When evaluating the eyes, there is less debate with regard to ideal esthetics, but they still can vary with ethnicity and current geographical fashion trends. In addition, when evaluating the eyes, there are some aspects of the analysis that can lead to the diagnosis of possible systemic disease. Furthermore, there are some other aspects of the analysis that are key to the preoperative evaluation to avoid postoperative complications.

Patient history and review of systems is particularly important when it comes to the eyes. Patients should be interviewed thoroughly in regards to eye problems including visual acuity, visual field issues, visual changes, eye irritation or dryness, and any use of artificial tears. For certain patients, it is ideal to obtain a thorough preoperative eye examination from an ophthalmologist or optometrist.

For some patients, simple visual acuity, visual field, and ocular motility tests can be performed in the office and documented. For patients with history of eye irritation or dry eyes, it is prudent to perform a tear secretion test. To perform

the tear secretion test, the eyes are anesthetized using Tetracaine topical anesthetic and then blotted dry. Next a Schirmer test strip is bent at the 5 mm mark and placed over the temporal palpebral conjunctiva, and patient instructed to look upward (with the lights dimmed).[19] The strip is left in place for 5 minutes and then removed. A normal Schirmer test will show 10 to 15 mm of wetting at 5 minutes.[19] Low secretion levels can lead to devastating results after cosmetic blepharoplasty. Low secretion levels are also seen with patient taking diuretics or antihistamines; thus, these patients may need to discontinue these medications to obtain an accurate reading.[19]

Assessment for lagophthalmus is an important part of the ocular examination, particularly for patients who have undergone eyelid or brow surgery in the past. This examination should be done by holding the brow in the proposed ideal position and asking the patient to close the eye gently. If lagophthalmus is noted preoperatively, caution is warranted with any surgical procedures that could potentiate the issue. The existence blepharoptosis should also be noted in such an examination, because correction of ptosis in such a patient will likely increase the degree of lagophthalmus.

In addition, testing for Bell's phenomenon is critical to avoid serious postoperative complications. Bell's phenomenon is tested for by having the patient tightly close their eyes, then the practitioner gently attempts to open the eyes. Upon opening the eyes, the position of the cornea and iris are noted. A normal response or "positive Bell's phenomenon" is demonstrated with the eye is observed elevating upward.[19] This response helps to protect the cornea from injury. Caution is warranted in patients without such a response as it could have deleterious side effects should they develop lagophthalmus postoperatively.

In youth, the ideal esthetic eye is seen with the lateral canthus 1 to 2 mm above the medial canthus, giving the eye a subtle lateral inclination (Fig. 7).[14] The typical vertical palpebral fissure height is 9 to 12 mm and horizontal palpebral fissure width is 28 to 30 mm. With aging, the horizontal palpebral fissure width decreases by approximately 10%.[20]

Upper eyelid

When evaluating the upper eyelid, it is key to assess them in conjunction with assessment of the brow position. In addition, the brow should be relaxed (or held in the position of the expected surgical brow lift) when examining the upper eyelid.

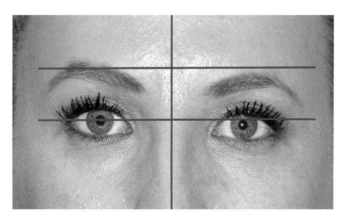

Fig. 6 Eyebrow asymmetry with orbital dystopia. Patient with asymmetrical eyebrow height and orbital dystopia.

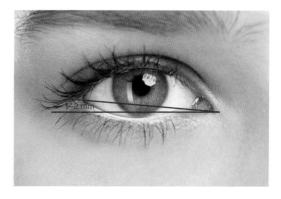

Fig. 7 The ideal esthetic eye. The ideal esthetic eye is seen with the lateral canthus located 1 to 2 mm higher than the medial canthus. This give the eye a subtle lateral inclination. (© shefkate / Adobe Stock.)

Surgical excision of upper eyelid skin can result in unmasking of preoperative brow ptosis, as with the excision of skin from the upper eyelid, the frontalis muscles is not needed to help improve the visual field anymore. The initial examination will be to assess the degree of excess skin and fat in the region. The degree of excess skin can be seen. One should understand and be able to differentiate between dermatochalasis and blepharochalasis. The former being the excess upper eyelid skin associated with aging, whereas the latter is excess skin from cyclic swelling edema and is typically seen in younger females.[19]

Excess or herniated fat should also be assessed at this time as well. This can be accomplished by pushing on the globe with gentle pressure (also called retropulsion), because the fat will protrude with the force applied to the globe.[1] In the upper eyelid, herniated fat is noted most commonly in the nasal fat pad. Any fullness laterally with such a maneuver is likely from prolapsed lacrimal gland and thus may require suspension back into lacrimal fossa at the time of surgery.

The marginal–reflex distance (MRD) and marginal crease distance (MCD) are key to evaluating the upper eyelid. The MRD is assessed ideally with the brow in a relaxed position and is the distance from the light reflex of the cornea to the upper eyelid margin at gaze in the primary position and measures 4 to 4.5 mm.[19]

When the MRD is within the normal range, the upper eyelid margin will typically be found resting in between the corneal limbus and edge of the iris or approximately 2 mm below the corneal limbus. When the MRD is less than normal, it is indicative of blepharoptosis. Blepharoptosis will not be corrected with a standard "skin excision only" blepharoplasty and requires adjunctive procedures to modify the levator palpebrae superioris and/or Muller's muscle. When the MRD is greater than normal, it considered eyelid retraction and could be a sign of thyroid eye disease, which should warrant further evaluation and management. Furthermore, thyroid eye disease and its retraction may still need to managed because even after management of the systemic disease, the eye disease may continue.[19]

If blepharoptosis is present and one wishes to correct it during blepharoplasty, evaluation of the levator palpebrae superioris and Muller's muscle function is important. One of the key components to upper eyelid position is function of the levator palpebrae superioris and Mueller's muscle. To assess levator function, one has the patient in the primary position at gaze and stabilizes the brow (to prevent movement caused by the frontalis) and then asks the patient to cycle between maximum upward gaze and downward gaze and ruler is used the measure the excursion of the eyelid margin. This excursion is normally 14 to 16 mm, and in patients with aponeurotic ptosis it is typically normal; if it is abnormal, it should prompt referral for further ptosis evaluation.[21] Evaluation of the Muller's muscle function requires instilling 2.5% phenylephrine drops in the eye and repeated at 3 to 5 minutes, if this results in 2 to 3 mm of eyelid elevation, it shows good Muller's muscle function and a Muller's muscle resection (via posterior approach) can be considered for ptosis repair.[21]

The upper eyelid crease is where the levator palpebrae superioris inserts into the orbicularis oculi. The MCD is the measurement from the upper eyelid crease to the eyelid margin at the central upper eyelid in the primary position and normally measures 9 to 11 mm (7-8 mm in men).[14,19] When the MCD is significantly greater than normal, one should suspect disinsertion of the levator aponeurosis, particularly when combined with ptosis of the upper eyelid.[19] When the MCD is significantly lower than normal, it typically requires reconstruction of the eyelid crease in conjunction with skin excision and possibly fat excision.[19] Altering of the crease height should always be discussed with the patient before surgery, because some patients may not be supportive of such alterations.[19]

Finally, when evaluating the upper eyelid, one should assess its volume. The stigmata of nonideal blepharoplasty is exemplified by the hollow appearance that can be seen from over-resection of muscle and fat and the resulting deep sulcus (Fig. 8). The upper eyelid in youth has an esthetic fullness to the lid–brow junction and its resulting convexity.[19] With aging, the upper eyelid and lid–brow junction becomes flat and even concave (Fig. 9). This volume loss can be accentuation with a blepharoplasty, which decreases the volume and can raise the eyelid crease further.[19] This result is an elongated MCD and increased exposure of pretarsal skin with deep hollow upper eyelid sulcus and volume depleted lid–brow junction. In such cases, preoperative analysis and diagnosis would prevent such results. When volume deficiency is noted, one may wish to consider a volume-enhancing blepharoplasty by leaving the orbicularis oculi intact and/or using a volumetric filler in the area.

Lower eyelid

Initial evaluation of the lower eyelid focuses on examination of the skin quality and quantity. In addition, one should evaluate for the presence of rhytids in the lower eyelid and cheek as well as lateral face in the areas of the crow's feet. The presence of significant rhytids in the area may require skin surface treatments (chemical peels or laser resurfacing) and/or neuromodulators to address areas of dynamic rhytids (like the crow's feet). In addition, attention should be focused on muscular aspects of the lower eyelid, particularly during smile, to assess for the presence of orbicularis hypertrophy, which may need to be addressed surgically with excision or with neuromodulators.

The lower eyelid is difficult to assess in isolation and needs to be assessed in conjunction with the midface. The midface

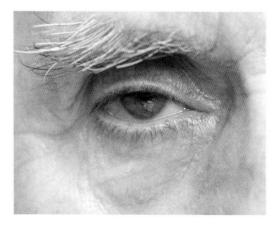

Fig. 8 Deep upper eyelid sulcus. As the levator palpebral superioris retreats into the orbit, the marginal crease distance increases, and the lid–brow junction volume decreases, it creates and accentuates the deep sulcus of the upper eyelid. (© Budimir Jevtic / Adobe Stock.)

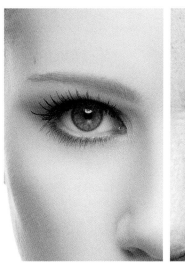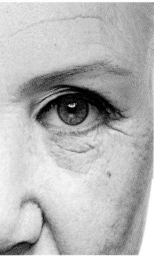

Fig. 9 Loss of volume from the upper eyelid. With age there is excess redundant skin of the upper eyelid with lateral hooding and decrease in volume in the area. (© JenkoAtaman / Adobe Stock.)

and lower eyelid blending are one of the key goals in restoring youthfulness in the area. In youth, in the profile view, the lower eyelid is a single mildly convex line and with age this line becomes elongated and a double convexity.[22]

Next, the volume in the area is important to assess. Volume assessment in the area involves assessment for excess or lack of volume. Excess volume can be seen in the lower eyelid in the form of orbicular hypertrophy and from herniated orbital fat. Assessment of orbicularis oculi hypertrophy is best assessed by having the patient smile or by squinting the eyes (Fig. 10). To assess for excess or herniated orbital fat, one can have the patient look in upward gaze while maintaining the head position and this will cause protrusion of the respective lower orbital fat pads. In addition, this can be accomplished by pushing on the globe with gentle pressure (also called retropulsion) and can help in the evaluation of fat in the area, because the fat will protrude with the force applied to the globe. The other areas of volume that can change with aging are descent of the midface and the apparent elongation of the lower eyelid with accentuation of the lower orbital rim. This is caused by descent of the midface, along with the associated fat pads, namely the suborbicularis oculi fat and the malar fat

pad. With these changes, the nasojugal groove (tear trough), orbitomalar crease, and nasolabial fold are accentuated. To obtain optimal outcome with blepharoplasty surgery, these changes need to corrected with suspension or camouflaged with fat repositioning or grafting.

The bony volume is also important because it provides support to structures of the midface and lower eyelid. Assessment for malar or orbital rim or tear tough bone atrophy or hypoplasia is key to optimizing surgical outcomes and ultimately patient expectations.

Lower eyelid position is particularly important for esthetic outcome of surgery and for prevention of postoperative complications. In the primary position at gaze, the lower eyelid will rest on the inferior corneal limbus. When the lower eyelid margin rest below the inferior corneal limbus it can be termed "excess scleral show." The etiology of scleral show can be multifactorial. The causes can be from midface hypoplasia or descent, lower eyelid laxity, postoperative complications, or as a manifestation of systemic disease like thyroid eye disease.

Lower eyelid laxity can be assessed by using the distraction test (Fig. 11) and the snap-back test (Fig. 12). To perform the lower lid distraction test (see Fig. 11), one grasps the lower eyelid gently in the center and distracts the eyelid anteriorly away from the globe; a distraction of less than 6 mm is normal[14] and greater than 6 mm is considered abnormal and should prompt consideration for additional permanent or temporary canthal support maneuvers (canthopexy, canthoplasty, orbicularis sling, or temporary lateral tarsorrhaphy). To perform the snap-back test (see Fig. 12), one pulls the lower eyelid inferiorly away from the globe and then releases the eyelid, a normal snap-back is shown when the eyelid returns to normal position before initiation of a blink.[23] A snap back test that does not have the eyelid return to normal position before blinking, is considered abnormal or "positive" and could signify an orbicularis defect and if the defect is noted unilaterally, one should consider further workup for possible facial nerve abnormality.[23] Lateral canthal integrity can be evaluation with nasal traction on the tendon and it should move minimally, if it move past the lateral limbus of the eye, tendon attenuation is likely.[19] Typically, laxity in the lower eyelid is a function of lack of lateral canthal support, the medial canthus should be

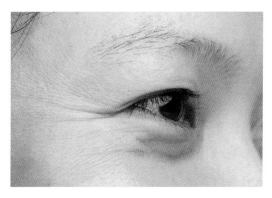

Fig. 10 Orbicularis hypertrophy. Upon smile and squinting of the eye, one can see the resulting dynamic rhytids in area of the crow's feeting and excess volume of the lower eyelid. (© rukxstockphoto / Adobe Stock.)

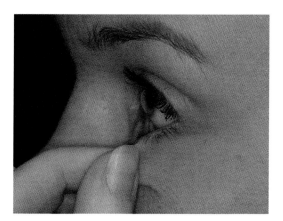

Fig. 11 Distraction test. To perform the lower lid distraction test, one grasps the lower eyelid gently in the center and distracts the eyelid anteriorly away from the globe, a distraction of less than 6 mm is normal[14] and greater than 6 mm is considered abnormal.

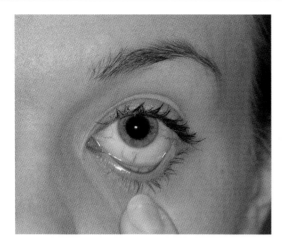

Fig. 12 Snap-back test. To perform the snap-back test, one pulls the lower eyelid inferiorly away from the globe and then releases the eyelid, a normal snap-back is shown when the eyelid returns to normal position before initiation of a blink.

considered as a possible etiology only if it moves greater than 2 mm upon traction.[14]

Summary

The world of cosmetic surgery is in constant flux and debate and is continually evolving. Thorough patient evaluation and review and discussion of the chief complaint are keys to success in cosmetic surgery. Detailed analysis and diagnosis before surgical intervention will lead better results and hopefully decreased incidence of complications. Following these guidelines will help one to maximize their success in the field.

References

1. Niamtu J 3rd. Cosmetic blepharoplasty. Atlas Oral Maxillofac Surg Clin North Am 2004;12(1):91–130.
2. Shapiro R. Principles and techniques used to create a natural hairline in surgical hair restoration. Facial Plast Surg Clin North Am 2004;12(2):201–17.
3. Shapiro R, Shapiro P. Hairline design and frontal hairline restoration. Facial Plast Surg Clin North Am 2013;21(3):351–62.
4. Pomerantz MA. Creating a hairline. Dermatol Clin 1999;17(2):271–5. vii; [discussion: 76].
5. Konior RJ, Simmons C. Patient selection, candidacy, and treatment planning for hair restoration surgery. Facial Plast Surg Clin North Am 2013;21(3):343–50.
6. Norwood OT. Patient selection, hair transplant design, and hairstyle. J Dermatol Surg Oncol 1992;18(5):386–94.
7. Sclafani AP. Aesthetic surgery of the forehead and upper third of the face: Thomas procedures in facial plastic surgery. Shelton (CT): People's Medical Pub. House-USA; 2011.
8. Han DS, Park JH. Aesthetic correction of a protrusive forehead through repositioning of the anterior wall of the frontal sinus. Archives of Craniofacial Surgery 2014;15(3):129–32.
9. Gunter JP, Antrobus SD. Aesthetic analysis of the eyebrows. Plast Reconstr Surg 1997;99(7):1808–16.
10. Westmore MG. Facial cosmetics in conjunction with surgery. Aesthetic Plastic Surgical Society Meeting. Vancouver (Canada), May 4–8, 1975.
11. Baker SB, Dayan JH, Crane A, et al. The influence of brow shape on the perception of facial form and brow aesthetics. Plast Reconstr Surg 2007;119(7):2240–7.
12. Hamamoto AA, Liu TW, Wong BJ. Identifying ideal brow vector position: empirical analysis of three brow archetypes. Facial Plast Surg 2013;29(1):76–82.
13. Yalcinkaya E, Cingi C, Soken H, et al. Aesthetic analysis of the ideal eyebrow shape and position. Eur Arch Otorhinolaryngol 2016;273(2):305–10.
14. Miloro M, Ghali GE, Larsen P, et al. Peterson's principles of oral and maxillofacial surgery. 2nd edition. Hamilton (Canada); London: B C Decker; 2004.
15. McKinney P, Mossie RD, Zukowski ML. Criteria for the forehead lift. Aesthetic Plast Surg 1991;15(2):141–7.
16. Connell BF, Lambros VS, Neurohr GH. The forehead lift: techniques to avoid complications and produce optimal results. Aesthetic Plast Surg 1989;13(4):217–37.
17. Matarasso A, Terino EO. Forehead-brow rhytidoplasty: reassessing the goals. Plast Reconstr Surg 1994;93(7):1378–89 [discussion: 90–1].
18. Haiavy J. Inland Cosmetic/Surgical Arts of Inland Empire - general cosmetic surgery fellowship. In: Dhaliwal H, editor. American Academy of Cosmetic Surgery; 2012-2013.
19. Fagien S, Putterman AM. Putterman's cosmetic oculoplastic surgery. 4th edition. Philadelphia: Saunders/Elsevier; 2008. p. 1. online resource (xiv, 347 p.).
20. van den Bosch WA, Leenders I, Mulder P. Topographic anatomy of the eyelids, and the effects of sex and age. Br J Ophthalmol 1999;83(3):347–52.
21. Martin JJ Jr. Ptosis repair in aesthetic blepharoplasty. Clin Plast Surg 2013;40(1):201–12.
22. Baker S, LaFerriere K, Larrabee WF Jr. Lower lid blepharoplasty: panel discussion, controversies, and techniques. Facial Plast Surg Clin North Am 2014;22(1):97–118.
23. De Silva DJ, Prasad A. Aesthetic canthal suspension. Clin Plast Surg 2015;42(1):79–86.

Botulinum Toxin Use in the Upper Face

Clement Qaqish, MD, DDS

KEYWORDS

- Botulinum toxin • Neurotoxin • Facial rhytids • Brow ptosis • IncobotulinumtoxinA • OnabotulinumtoxinA
- Lateral canthal rhytids

KEY POINTS

- Botulinum toxin is a potent exotoxin that disrupts neuromuscular transmission by inhibiting the release for acetylcholine from the presynaptic membrane resulting in attenuation of muscle contraction.
- There are 3 formulations of Botulinum toxin A approved for cosmetic use in the United States: onabotulinumtoxinA (Botox), incobotulinumtoxinA (Xeomin), and abobotulinumtoxinA (Dysport).
- All 3 products are US Food and Drug Administration approved for the reduction of dynamic glabellar rhytids with the exception of Botox, which is also approved for the treatment of mimetic lateral canthal rhytids. Much of its use is off-label.
- Most complications can be avoided with knowledge of the functional anatomy of the upper face as well as proper injection technique. Some of the more serious complications include brow and/or eyelid ptosis and diplopia.
- The administration of neurotoxin has evolved to become individualized. More sophisticated injection techniques have allowed the clinician to sculpt the brow in a favorable fashion while preserving animation.

Introduction

The nonsurgical treatment of the aging face is centered on identifying the cause of changes to the quality and texture of skin as well as the volume deficiencies in the dermis and underlying tissue. Hyperdynamic rhytids, particularly in the facial upper third, not only can be visually undesirable but, over time, also can result in dermal atrophy and corresponding static facial rhytids. These changes, in concert with dermal photoaging, contribute to the stigmata of the aging face.

Since the introduction of botulinum toxin (BoNT) for the reduction of glabellar rhytids in 1992 and the corresponding US Food and Drug Administration (FDA) approval of the neurotoxin for this therapeutic indication over a decade later, the use of neurotoxins or neuromodulators for cosmetic purposes has seen unprecedented growth.[1] In fact, between 2000 and 2014, there has been a 700-fold increase in the number of annual injections.[2] According to data from the American Association of Plastic Surgeons, there were 6.3 million cosmetic neurotoxin injections performed in the United States in 2013.[2] BoNT injections remain the most common nonsurgical cosmetic treatment for facial rhytids worldwide.

BoNT is an exotoxin, produced by the obligate anaerobe *Clostridium botulinum*, a spore-forming gram-positive rod found in the soil. The toxin causes the disease Botulism, a form of food poisoning that is quite rare today because heating destroys the toxin and because the addition of nitrates to processed meats prevents the growth of the bacteria.[3,4] Several serotypes of the toxin are produced by the bacteria with types A, B, and E being known to cause disease in humans.[3,5] The toxin is a dimeric protein that acts at the neuromuscular junction (NMJ). It binds to the presynaptic membrane of the NMJ and enters the terminal neuron via receptor-mediated endocytosis.[4,5] The acidic environment within the endosome cleaves the complex into its active metabolites.[5] The net effect is irreversible inhibition of acetylcholine release and decreased contraction of the motor unit. With ongoing turnover of the NMJ, however, contractile function returns after several weeks, which correlates with the return of pretreatment muscle strength, 3 to 4 months after injection.[3,4]

BoNT is currently used for several conditions in which the desired result is relaxation or even paralysis of targeted musculature. It has been used to treat a variety of conditions, including strabismus, blepharospasm, hemifacial spasm, dystonia, hyperhydrosis, headache, and facial wrinkling.[1,3,5–8] Novel therapeutic uses are continuously being reported across a spectrum of medical specialties. Its use in cosmetic medicine lies in the denervation of the mimetic muscles of facial expression, thereby reducing the pull of these muscles on the overlying skin. The net effect is temporary reduction in the appearance of dynamic lines.

Preoperative planning and pretreatment assessment

Product selection

There are currently 3 formulations of BoNT commercially available that are FDA approved for cosmetic use: onabotulinum-toxin A (onaBoNT-A, Botox; Allergan Inc, Irvine, CA, USA), abobotulinum-toxin A (aboBoNT-A, Dysport; Galderma Laboratories, LP, Fortworth, TX, USA), and incobotulinum-toxin A (incoBoNT-A, Xeomin; Merz Pharmaceuticals, LLC, Greensboro, NC, USA). All formulations are FDA approved for the treatment of globular rhytids in patients 18 to 65.[9–11] However, onaBoNT

The author has nothing to disclose.

Private Practice, San Diego Surgical Arts, 10672 Wexford Street, Suite 270, San Diego, CA 92131, USA

E-mail address: drq@sdsurgicalarts.com

1061-3315/16/$ - see front matter © 2016 Elsevier Inc. All rights reserved.
http://dx.doi.org/10.1016/j.cxom.2016.05.006
oralmaxsurgeryatlas.theclinics.com

(Botox) is the only product with additional FDA approval for the treatment of lateral canthal lines.[9] Rimabotulinum-toxin B (RimaBoNT-B, Mybloc; Soltice Neurosciences Inc, San Francisco, CA, USA) is FDA approved for the treatment of cervical dystonia. This product is also used off label in nonresponders to serotype A of the toxin.

Variations between the 3 commercially available products in potency, onset time, therapeutic duration, and immunogenicity are not significant.[12] It should be noted that unit dosing for all BoNT-A formulations is not interchangeable, and therapeutic endpoints are achieved with different unit doses— most notably between aboBoNT-A (Dysport) and the other 2 serotypes.[4,12] Botox and Xeomin are dosed in comparable unit values, whereas Dysport requires 2.5 to 3 times of its own unit value (Speywood units) to achieve the same clinical result.[12]

Product storage

All commercially available BoNT-A products are stored as a lyophilized powder in a vacuum-sealed container. Both Botox and Dysport are shipped in dry ice and require storage in temperatures between 2°C and 8°Cwith a stable shelf life at this temperature of 2 to 3 years.[9,11] Xeomin, however, has a stable shelf of 3 years at temperatures ranging from −20°C to 25°C and therefore does not require refrigeration for shipment.[10] All 3 products, however, require refrigerated storage between 2°C and 8°Cafter they are reconstituted, for use in patients. Although all neurotoxin vials are marketed and labeled for single use within 24 hours of reconstitution, most clinicians store reconstituted product for significantly longer periods of time. In fact, a general consensus exists that product refrigerated at 2°C to 8°C can be effective for up to 6 weeks.[13,14] There are some investigators who advocate freezing the product after reconstitution to allow it to retain its potency for up to 6 months.[13]

Product dilution

Product dilution is an area of frequent controversy. Toxin concentrations vary among treating clinicians, area used, and indication. Patient preference also has some impact on the concentration of neurotoxin used. The author prefers a more dilute mixture and corresponding decreased dose of neuromodulator for cosmetic use because it provides what is thought to be a softer look. For treatment of dystonias and in patients with more pronounced dynamic rhytids, the author uses more concentrated product. Theoretically, a less concentrated (greater diluent) product carries with it a greater risk of diffusion or more appropriately spread, and the potential for complications, and inadequate therapeutic outcomes. However, this has shown not to be the case.[15,16] Recommended product dilutions are shown in Table 1. All manufacturers recommend reconstitution with preservative-free normal saline; however, most clinicians seem to agree that preserved saline is a preferred diluent because the 0.9% benzyl alcohol appears to impart a mild analgesic effect without compromising the product potency or longevity.[17] Diluent is drawn up in a 3-mL syringe and a blunt-tip needle. The needle is then used to pierce the stopper of the product vial, and most of the saline is taken up automatically by vacuum pressure (Fig. 1), with the need for only gentle pressure to push the remainder of the diluent into the vial. The reconstituted mixture is then rolled to gently dissolve the product. Several investigators

Table 1 Type and concentration of botulinum toxin	
Product Toxin	Concentration (units/mL)
Dysport 300-unit vial	
1.5 mL	20/0.1
3 mL	10/0.1
Botox 100-unit vial	
2.5 mL	4/0.1
5 mL	2/0.1[a]
Xeomin 100-unit vial	
2.5 mL	4/0.1
5 mL	2/0.1[a]

Sample dilutions of different BoNT products.
[a] Denotes a dilute mixture often used by the author in the forehead and occasionally the glabella to impart a softer look to treatment, resulting in an appreciable preservation of animation while blunting mimetic lines.

advise against vigorously shaking the vial because this could create foaming and decrease its potency. Other investigators have found this not to be true. Because Xeomin is stored as an actual powder, Merz Pharmaceuticals recommends inverting the cap while reconstituting the product to ensure any leftover product under the cap is dissolved.[10] Missing this step in the reconstitution of incoBoNT-A may be a reason for the anecdotal reports of Xeomin having a decreased duration of action when compared with Botox. Indicated volume of product is drawn up using a 1-mm Luer-Lock syringe and a 20-gauge needle, and then a 33-gauge 0.5-inch needle (Sterjet needle; TSK Laboratories, Tochigi-Ken, Japan) is used to inject the product (Fig. 2). Some investigators advocate the use of a 31-gauge diabetic syringe (hubless needle and attached syringe) to both draw up product from vial and inject patients.[3] The author feels that, while this technique ensures less waste of product, for multiple injection sites, the needle on a diabetic syringe blunts quickly, producing more injection site pain. For most injections in the upper face (with the exception of heavy dynamic glabellar rhytids), the author uses a concentration of 2 unit/0.1 mL or 20 units in a 1-mL Luer-Lock syringe. For more pronounced hyperdynamic rhytids and in patients insistent on

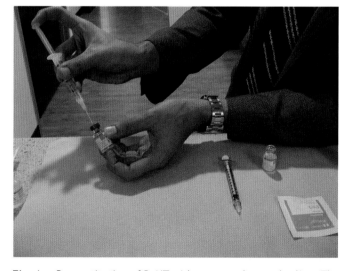

Fig. 1   Reconstitution of BoNT with preserved normal saline. The vacuum seal within the vial draws up the diluent automatically.

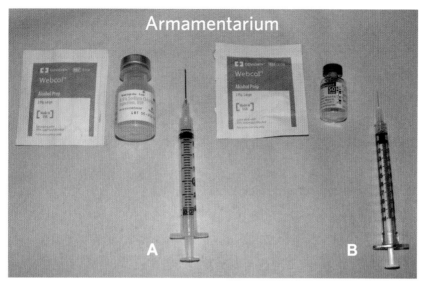

Fig. 2 Armamentarium for reconstitution and injection of BoNT. (*A*) Normal saline drawn up in 3-mL syringe and blunt 21-gauge needle shown in (*A*). (*B*) Luer-Lock 1-mL syringe and 33-gauge needle used to inject product. (Medtronic, Minneapolis, MN.)

no residual muscle movement, the author uses the recommended 4 units/0.1 mL concentration (see Table 1).

Physical examination and patient education

Despite the plethora of information disseminated on the Web, television, and print ads, most patients seeking neuromodulator treatment are largely unaware of how the product works and certainly the limitations of the product. In the author's practice, all new cosmetic patients fill out a detailed medical history and a brief questionnaire about the patient's experience with cosmetic procedures. There are few contraindications to neuromodulator treatment, and most are relative contraindications. BoNT is a category C medication for both pregnancy and lactation, and the author will not inject pregnant or actively breast-feeding patients.[9–11] Patients with neuromuscular disorders, such as amyotrophic lateral sclerosis, myasthenia gravis, Eaton-Lambert syndrome, and the motor neuron diseases, can theoretically be worsened by administration of neurotoxin and are therefore not suitable candidates for neurotoxin treatment.[9–11] Patients taking medications that can interfere with neuromuscular transmission should be avoided because they may enhance the paralytic effect of the toxin (Box 1).[4,6] Patients with known hypersensitivity to the ingredients in the product (albumin, sodium chloride, milk protein in the case of Dysport or the toxin itself) should also be avoided.[6,18] Relative contraindications include any anticoagulation therapy. In fact, patients are asked, where appropriate, to discontinue nonsteroidal anti-inflammatory drugs (NSAIDs) and aspirin use 2 weeks before treatment to avoid excessive bruising. A final relative contraindication relates to the patient's understanding of what can realistically be achieved by the product.

New patients to nonsurgical cosmetic facial treatments are asked, with mirror in hand, to point out lines that bother them. Any asymmetries that are readily apparent should be pointed out to the patient and documented. Patients are often more critical and will scrutinize their treated appearance much more than before treatment. Although the author does not routinely use photodocumentation for

neuromodulator patients, it can certainly be of value, particularly when neurotoxin treatment is combined with other modalities like facial fillers and/or resurfacing procedures. If there are mimetic lines in the glabella, forehead, or lateral canthal region, the patient is informed that neuromodulator treatment alone can help ameliorate this concern. Often, however, there are corresponding static lines that are often made worse and invariably caused by the repetitive action of the muscles of facial expression. The presence of combined static and mimetic rhytids requires a discussion about the need for combination therapy to either volumize or resurface the skin in addition to blunting the muscles of facial expression with a neuromodulator. The synergy created by combination therapy is often what is needed to meet patient expectations about wrinkle reduction. Through a knowledge and understanding of the anatomy of the muscles of facial expression in the periocular region and forehead and through the use of selective chemodenervation, neurotoxin use in wrinkle reduction has become much more sophisticated than it once was. The arguably undesirable "frozen appearance" imparted by treatment can be avoided by the selective targeting of brow depressors and elevators, and in the author's opinion, by limiting the dose.

Box 1. Medications interfering with neuromuscular transmissions

- Antibiotics (certain aminoglycosides, lincosamides, polymyxins)
- Penicillamine
- Quinine
- Calcium channel blockers
- Neuromuscular-blocking agents (atracurium, succinylocholine)
- Anticholinesterases
- Magnesium sulfate
- Quinidine

Modest lifting and sculpting of the brow can be achieved while still preserving facial animation.[19,20]

Procedural technique

Patient preparation and positioning

Alcohol pads are used to wipe injection sites to remove facial oils and makeup. Some advocate more intensive cleansing before treatment with chlorhexidine scrub,[3] but this is not the practice of the author. Topical anesthetics are rarely used before treatment; however, ice packs have been shown to be beneficial in reducing discomfort both immediately before and immediately after injection. Although there are is no evidence to support a specific position of the patient, the author prefers the patient semireclined, supported by a headrest, for comfort. The nondominant hand is used to palpate pertinent anatomic landmarks where appropriate. Injection should be slow and perpendicular to a noncontracted muscle or subcutaneously. Although some investigators may advocate a bolus injection and massage, the current author uses a serial puncture application (Fig. 3).

Technique

The muscles of facial expression insert directly onto the undersurface of the skin. Repetitive contraction therefore causes characteristic rhytids to form perpendicular to the direction or vector of contraction (Fig. 4). Selective chemodenervation of the upper nasal area ("bunny lines"), glabella ("11's"), forehead, and lateral canthal area ("crow's feet") can help blunt these hyperdynamic lines, softening the appearance of the upper face. BoNT is administered in "units." One unit of BoNT-A represents the lethal dose in 50% of a group of Swiss Webster mice within 3 days of intraperitoneal injection.[4,15] Extrapolated to a 70-kg person, the median lethal dose is estimated to be between 2500 and 3000 units. Although the exact dose of toxin known to cause toxicity in unknown, it is generally agreed that single doses of BoNT-A should not exceed 500 units.[8]

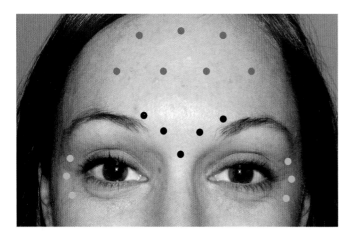

Fig. 3 Sample injection points for this patient. Black lines denote classic glabellar injection points. Blue points denote injection points for this patient's forehead, whose length requires 2 rows of injections in the author's view. Green lines denote the injection pattern in the lateral canthal region.

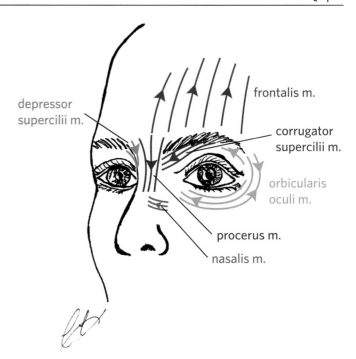

Fig. 4 Colored arrows represent regions of the muscles of facial expression, specifically the brow elevators and depressors. Arrow direction indicates direction of contraction and pull on the brow or associated tissue. The mimetic lines created by muscle contraction are perpendicular to these colored arrows. m., muscle.

This amount is well above the typical dose administered for cosmetic purposes.

Glabella

Prominent glabellar furrows can unintentionally project worry, anger, and advanced age and are often thought by patients to be undesirable. The glabellar region contains the medial brow depressors, which include the corrugators, procerus, supramedial orbicular oculi, and the variably present depressor supercilii.[4–6] The treatment of glabellar rhytids focuses on the attenuation of mainly the procerus and corrugator supercilii. Contraction of the corrugators as well as both the depressor supercilii and the medial orbicularis oculi produces the vertical dynamic lines between the eyebrows or the "11's." The procerus and depressor supercilii produce the horizontal lines over the bridge of the nose when contracted (see Fig. 4). Product inserts for both Botox and Xeomin recommend 5 injection points—2 in the corrugators bilaterally and one in the procerus with a recommended dose of approximately 20 units and a concentration of 4 units/ 0.1 mL.[9,10] Although this standard dosage is still commonly used and may serve as a guide to the novice injector, many clinicians, including the author, have moved to tailoring injection points and dosage to the individual. Considerations should be made to muscle strength, anatomy (rhytid pattern), baseline asymmetries as well as patient desires when deciding on dose and injection pattern. The frozen look is no longer a desirable therapeutic outcome for most, and lower dosages in this region can blunt undesirable furrows while maintaining some movement and expression. Care should be taken when injecting this area to stay at least 1 cm from the superior orbital rim and inject perpendicular to the muscle belly or

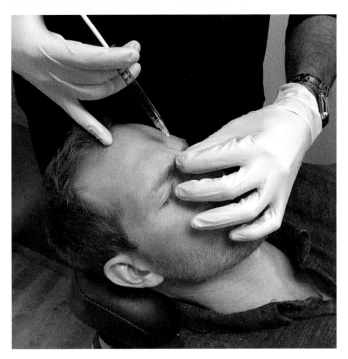

Fig. 5 Injection technique for the glabella is shown. The author's preference is to directly inject the bellies of the corrugators and procerus when injecting the glabella. Subcutaneous injection is also acceptable and preferable in other areas such as the lateral canthal area.

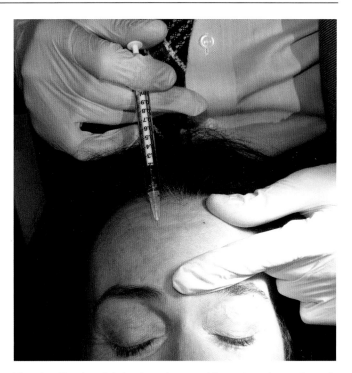

Fig. 6 Forehead injection shown with patient intermittently animating and with injection point at least 2.5 cm above the supraorbital rim.

subcutaneously (Fig. 5). This method reduces the risk of spread of the product, permeation of the orbital septum, and paralysis of the levator palpebrae superioris, which may cause upper eyelid ptosis.[6,8]

Forehead

Although the injection of the forehead may afford more "real estate," a thorough knowledge of the anatomy of the frontalis (the lone brow elevator) and its relationship with the brow depressors is imperative. The frontalis is a muscle whose twin bellies are often divided by a central tendinous attachment. As a result, midline injections may not be required in certain patients. The muscle originates from the galea aponeurosis and inserts into the frontal bone brow complex and interdigitates with the brow depressors. The lateral extent of the muscle is the temporal fusion line, a bony landmark that can be palpated.[4] Contraction of the muscle produces the characteristic horizontal rhytids. Care must be taken in the evaluation and correction of these furrows because isolated treatment may unmask a true eyelid or brow ptosis. The goal of treatment is to soften undesirable lines without causing brow ptosis or eliminate all expressiveness from the upper face. Several investigators advocate injection above the midline of the forehead, whereas others use a measurement of 2.5 to 3 cm above the orbital rim to avoid brow ptosis (Fig. 6). The author never injects the forehead in isolation. The glabellar complex and forehead are almost always injected simultaneously. Typical dosing for the forehead varies between 10 and 25 units of BoNT A depending on forehead length and strength of muscle activity.

Brow contouring

Understanding the functional anatomy of the muscles of facial expression in the periocular region can aid in manipulating brow position and contour. Skillfully balancing the opposing effects of the antagonistic muscles with neurotoxin can help elevate and selectively sculpt the brow, whose resting position is dictated by a balance between the depressors and lone brow elevator (frontalis). Preferential chemodenervation of the glabellar complex (corrugator supercilii, procerus, depressor supercilii, and medial orbicular oculi) can produce as much as a 2-mm medial brow elevation.[19–21] Lateral brow elevation can be achieved by injecting the superolateral orbicularis oculi immediately beneath the desired area of elevation. Care must be taken with this technique to keep injection away from orbital rim in a superior direction (Fig. 7). Injecting too high in this area may result in neurotoxin spread to the inferior frontalis and paradoxical brow ptosis.

Lateral canthal lines

Lateral canthal wrinkling (crow's feet) may represent one of the earliest signs of aging. Hyperdynamic rhytids in the lateral periorbital region are created by the contraction of the orbicular oculi. It is a sphincter muscle that is circumferentially oriented. Contraction, with squinting or smiling, produces wrinkles that extend radially from the lateral canthus (Fig. 8A). Injection in this area should be tailored to wrinkle pattern; however, injections should be superficial, producing a characteristic wheal 1 cm away from the orbital rim and 1.5 cm away from the lateral canthus to avoid spread of product to unwanted areas. A total dose of 10 to 30 units

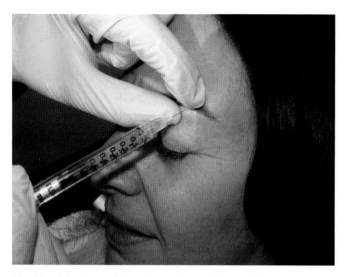

Fig. 7 Injection of 2 units in the infralateral brow region to attenuate the supralateral orbicularis oculi in hopes of achieving lateral brow elevation. Injection is superficial, immediately beneath intended area of elevation.

can be given typically divided among 2 to 3 injection sites per side (Fig. 8B). The author typically injects 3 sites per side, with one injection on the same horizontal plane as the lateral canthus and 2 other injections flanking the canthal injections. Wrinkle pattern sometimes requires modification of this pattern. Again, treatment should be individualized. Dosage is dependent on depth and extent of hyperdynamic rhytids. Care should be taken not to inject too far inferiorly. Injection of the zygomaticus may affect upper lip tone, resulting in an upper lip asymmetry.[22] Injection medial to the midpupillary line should be avoided because of the potential risk of ectropion and epiphora.[8] It should be noted that some clinicians perform infralid injections in patients who desire enlargement of the palpebral aperture. This

procedure should be avoided in patients with any lower lid laxity whatsoever, and a pretreatment snap test should be performed to evaluate lower eyelid tone. If infralid injections are attempted, care should be taken to ensure injections are very superficial and at least 2 mm below the ciliary margin.[23]

Transverse nasal rhytids

Animation of the periocular region can create wrinkling in the lateral nasal sidewall. These "bunny lines" are the result of contraction of the transverse portion of the nasalis muscle (see Fig. 4). One to 4 units can be injected per side with care taken to palpate for and avoid the angular artery, which tracks superiorly in this region.

Complications

Although not considered true complications, there are several undesirable sequelae of neuromodulator treatment. Injection site pain, needle marks, edema, bruising, hematoma, and mild erythema are all commonly observed with treatment.[4,6,9,10,15] Earlier onset of action of one anatomic site over another occurs commonly as well and is not necessarily a complication. Injection site pain can be minimized using smaller-gauged needles. The author uses 33-gauge needles for injection. The use of preserved saline with benzyl alcohol has an analgesic effect during injection.[17] Icing immediately before injection dulls the skin and has the added benefit of causing local vasoconstriction to help minimize vessel puncture and bruising. Bleeding can also be minimized with more superficial injecting. Patients on NSAIDs and anticoagulants are asked to discontinue medication, if permissible, 7 to 10 days before injection. Bleeding or hematoma can be managed fairly easily with direct pressure and ice.

The most notable and alarming complications are regional, where neurotoxin spread is beyond its intended therapeutic area and neuromuscular blockade of unintended adjacent sites

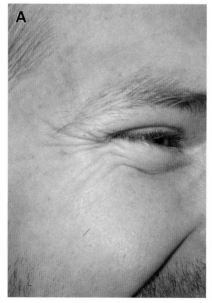
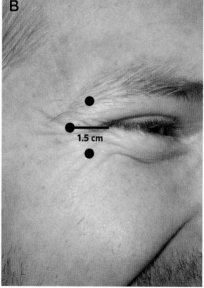

Fig. 8 (A) Lateral canthal rhytids in a 34-year-old Caucasian man. (B) Black dots denote injection points, with the middle injection positioned at least 1.5 cm from the lateral canthus, and all injection points at least 1 cm from the palpable orbital rim.

is seen. For example, too inferior of an injection in the lateral canthal area resulting in chemodenervation of the zygomaticus muscle can create an upper lip asymmetry.[6,22,24] Brow ptosis is a potential complication of forehead injections or improperly placed glabellar injections. Preservation of the function of the inferior frontalis muscle 2 to 3 cm superior to the supraorbital rim is imperative to preserving brow position. Management is centered on ensuring denervation of the antagonistic brow depressors. If this was done as part of original treatment, then management is expectant. Periocular injection too close to the orbital rim may result in untoward spread toward the orbital septum and denervation of the levator palpebrae superioris, resulting in upper eyelid ptosis.[6,22,25] Iatrogenic ptosis can be managed with the use of topical apraclonidine 0.5% drops (Iopidine; Alcon Laboratories Inc, Ft. Worth, TX, USA) 3 times per day, until symptoms resolve. Iopidine is an α-2-adrenergic agonist that stimulates the sympathetically innervated Mueller muscle, stimulation of which can cause as much as a 2-mm elevation in the ptotic eyelid. Overzealous inject of the lower orbicularis oculi may result in spread of the toxin to within the orbit and possible attenuation of the lateral or inferior rectus muscles with resultant diplopia.[22] Progressive diplopia after injection warrants an ophthalmologic consultation, although management is largely expectant.

Since the reduction in complexing protein content of the solution in the late 1990s, there have been no reports of anaphylaxis to BoNT injection.[4] Allergy to any of the components of the preparations is possible, but reported reactions are limited to rare rashes and granuloma formation.[6,25] Nonresponders to primary treatment are also quite rare. Improper dosing and product degradation are far more likely explanations that should be ruled out if product does not appear to be working. A secondary nonresponse or a dramatically decreased effect may be the result of immune desensitization. The neurotoxin represents a foreign protein load that, in theory, could trigger an immunologic response producing blocking antibodies. The development of antibodies seems to correlate with the number of injections, frequency of treatment, and total cumulative dose.[18,26] Limiting injections to less than 400 units over a 3-month period appears to negate the development of a detectable humoral response.[18] Should immunologic resistance develop to BoNT-A, BoNT-B (Myobloc) may be used as an alternative. Distal spread of the toxin and systemic botulism is a theoretical concern but has not been reported with the doses and injection sites typically used for cosmetic purposes.[27]

After procedure care

There are a plethora of recommendations about after procedure management of patients receiving neurotoxin. Some

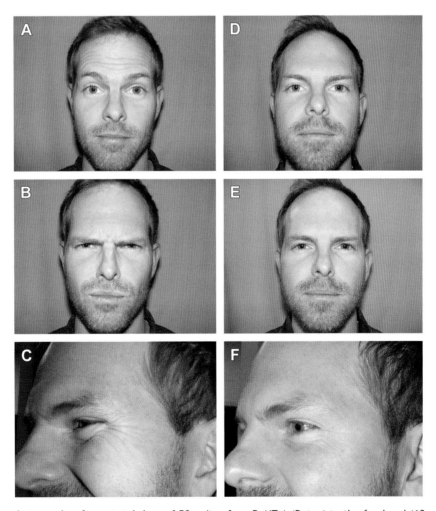

Fig. 9 Before and after photographs after a total dose of 50 units of onaBoNT-A (Botox) to the forehead (18 units), glabella (18 units), and lateral canthal areas (14 units). (*A–C*) Pretreatment photos. (*D–F*) Five days after treatment.

clinicians instruct patients to animate there face vigorously to increase uptake of toxin. Others advocate massage of the injected area for similar reasons. Recommendations on after procedure activity limitations are also varied. None of these recommendations have been shown to improve outcomes or decrease complications. Recovery from the procedure is very rapid, with the fluid wheals dissolving within 15 minutes of injection. The author recommends that patients remain upright and avoid vigorous exercise for 4 hours to theoretically reduce the spread of toxin to unwanted areas. Typically, peak effect is seen by 14 days,[9,10] which is when patients are asked to follow-up for re-evaluation and touch-ups, if necessary. Repeat injections past 3 weeks should be avoided because it becomes difficult to determine whether more neurotoxin is needed or the muscle activity observed represents a wearing off of previously injected product. Patients are typically reappointed between 3 to 4 months for additional treatment.

Outcomes

The outcomes of experienced injectors (with proper injection technique and knowledge of the functional anatomy of the face) of BoNT either as monotherapy or, in combination with other therapeutic modalities, are excellent (Fig. 9). Patient dissatisfaction stems from a lack understanding of the limitations of the product in wrinkle reduction and a failure to understand what can realistically be achieved with chemodenervation—which does not address static rhytids, volume loss, and other manifestations of photodamage. Minor complaints about known sequelae of the procedure, such as injection site pain, bruising, and swelling, may be upsetting to uninformed patients. Proper patient education, through informed consent, will help prevent the need for explanation, as though it were an excuse, if one of these undesirable events were to occur.

Summary

The use of BoNT for therapeutic purposes has revolutionized medicine. New therapeutic applications of the neurotoxin are constantly being reported. Its use in cosmetic medicine, particularly for facial rejuvenation, has evolved from its cookie-cutter approach of all or nothing chemodenervation, to a sculpting of the brow and forehead complex with preservation of facial animation. A thorough understanding of the functional anatomy of the muscles of facial expression as well as intimate product knowledge will enable the clinician to deliver optimal esthetic results.

References

1. Carruthers JA, Carruthers JA. Treatment of glabellar frown lines C. Botulinum-A exotoxin. J Dermatol Surg Oncol 1992;18:17—21.
2. The American Society for Aesthetic Plastic Surgery (ASAPS) 2013 facts and statistics report. Available at: http://www.surgery.org/sites/default/files/2014-Stats.pdf. Accessed December 15, 2015.
3. Erickson BP, Lee WW, Cohen J, et al. The role of neurotoxins in the periorbital and mid facial areas. Facial Plast Surg Clin North Am 2015;23:243—55.
4. Matarasso A, Shafer D. Botulinum toxin injections for facial rejuvenation. In: Nahai F, editor. The art of aesthetic surgery: principles and techniques. 2nd edition. St Louis (MO): Quality Medical Publishing; 2011. p. 243—6.
5. Feily A, Fallahi H, Zandian D, et al. A succinct review of botulinum toxin in dermatology; update of cosmetic and non-cosmetic use. J Cosmet Dermatol 2011;10(1):58—67.
6. Klein AW. Contraindications and complications with the use of botulinum toxin. Clin Dermatol 2004;22(1):66—75.
7. Matarasso A, Centeon RF, Boswell CB. Botulinum toxin for management of focal hyperhidrosis. Aesthet Surg J 2002;23: 67—9.
8. Sorensen EP, Urman C. Cosmetic complications: rare and serious events following botulinum toxin and soft tissue filler administration. J Drugs Dermatol 2015;14(5):486—91.
9. Botox Cosmetic (2014) OnabotulinumtoxinA: full prescribing information. Allergan Inc., Irvine.
10. Xeomin (2013) IncobotulinumtoxinA: full prescribing information. Merz Pharmaceuticals, LLC, Greensboro.
11. Dysport (2010) AbobotulinumtoxinA: full prescribing information. Medicis Aesthetics Inc., Scottsdale.
12. Chen JJ, Dashtipour K. Abo-, inco-, ona-, and rimabotulinum toxins in clinical therapy: a primer. Pharmacotherapy 2013;33(3): 304—18.
13. Liu A, Carruthers A, Cohen JL, et al. Recommendations and current practices for reconstitution and storage of botulinum toxin type A. J Am Acad Dermatol 2012;67:373—8.
14. Hui JI, Lee WW. Efficacy of fresh versus refrigerated botulinum toxin in the treatment of lateral periorbital rhytids. Ophthal Plast Recontr Surg 2007;23(6):433—8.
15. Lowe NJ, Shah A, Lowe PL, et al. Dosing, efficacy and safety plus the use of computerized photography for botulinum toxins type A for upper facial lines. J Cosmet Laser Ther 2010;12: 106—11.
16. Carruthers A, Carruthers J, Cohen J. Dilution volume of botulinum toxin type A for the treatment of glabellar rhytids: does it matter? Dermatol Surg 2007;33:S97—104.
17. Carruthers J, Fagien S, Mattarasso SL, et al. Consensus recommendations on the use of botulinum toxin type A in facial esthetics. Plast Reconstr Surg 2004;114:1S—22S.
18. Jankovic J. Botulinum toxin: clinical implications of antigenicity and immunoresistance. In: Brin MF, Jankovic J, Hallet M, editors. Scientific and therapeutic aspects of botulinum toxin. Philadelphia: Lippencott Williams and Wilkins; 2002. p. 409—15.
19. Huang W, Rogashefsky AS, Foster JA. Browlift with botulinum toxin. Dermatol Surg 2000;26:55—60.
20. Frankel AS, Kamer FM. Chemical browlift. Arch Otolaryngol Head Neck Surg 1998;124:3221—3.
21. Prager W, Huber-Vorlander J, Taufig AZ, et al. Botulinum toxin type A treatment in the upper face: retrospective analysis of daily practice. Clin Cosmet Investig Dermatol 2012;5:53—8.
22. Matarasso A, Matarasso SL. Treatment guidelines for botulinum toxin type A for peri-ocular injection and a report of upper lip ptosis following injections of lateral canthal rhytids. Plast Reconstr Surg 2001;108:208—14.
23. Flynn TC, Carruthers JA, Carruthers JA. Botulinum toxin treatment of lower eyelid improves infra-lid rhytids and widens the eye. Dermatol Surg 2001;27:703—8.
24. Carruthers J, Carruthers A. Botulinum toxin in facial rejuvenation: an update. Dermatol Clin 2009;27(4):417—25.
25. Klein AW. Complications, adverse reactions, and insights with the use of botulinum toxin. Dermatol Surg 2003;29:549—56.
26. Goschel H, Wolfarth K, Frevert J, et al. Botulinum A toxin therapy. Neutralizing and non-neutralizing antibodies-therapeutic consequences. Exp Neurol 1997;147:96—102.
27. Crowner BE, Torres-Rusotto D, Carter AP, et al. Systemic weakness after therapeutic injections of botulinum toxin A: a case series and review of the literature. Clin Neuropharmacol 2010; 33(5):243—7.

Further readings

Carruthers A, Carruthers J, Said S. Dose ranging study of botulinum toxin type A in the treatment of glabellar rhytids. Dermatol Surg 2005;32(4):414—22.

Cartee TV, Monheit GD. An overview of botulinum toxins: past, present and future. Clin Plast Surg 2011;38:409—26.

Flynn TC. Botulinum toxin: examining duration of effect in facial esthetic applications. Am J Clin Dermatol 2010;11(3):183—99.

Guyuron B, Tucker T, Kriegler J. Botulinum toxin and migraine surgery. Plast Reconstr Surg 2003;112(5):171S—3S.

Hsu TS, Dover JS, Arndt KA. Effect of volume and concentration on the diffusion of botulinum exotoxin A. Arch Dermatol 2004;140(11):1351—4.

Matarasso SL. Complications of botulinum exotoxin for hyperfunctional lines. Dermatol Surg 1998;24:1249—54.

Injectable Fillers in the Upper Face

Jacob Haiavy, MD, DDS [a],*, Husam Elias, MD, DMD [b]

KEYWORDS

- Upper facial rejuvenation • Facial fillers • Autologous fat grafting • Fat transfer • Perioorbital rejuvenation
- Facial aging

KEY POINTS

- Facial fillers are valuable in volumetric rejuvenation of the upper face, alone, or as an adjunct to cosmetic surgical facial procedures and neurotoxins. The injector must evaluate the need of the patient and select the appropriate filler for specific anatomic area.
- HA fillers are considered the workhorse of volumetric facial enhancement owing to simplicity of use, limited adverse effects, and reversibility.
- Autologous fat grafting is gaining more popularity with long-term predictable results.
- Choice of facial filler is a shared decision between the patient and the surgeon. It is important for the facial surgeon to familiarize himself or herself with different types of existing facial fillers to choose the right material for the right anatomic area.

 Video content accompanies this article at http://www.oralmaxsurgeryatlas.theclinics.com.

Introduction

Over the past few decades, it has become clear that facial aging is a complex 3-dimensional process that involves all tissue planes and results in cutaneous changes, muscle laxity, fat atrophy and loss of volume, as well as bone loss in certain parts of the face. Aging in the upper face, like aging in the remainder of the face, is affected by genetics, loss of volume, and loss of support over time. In addition, extrinsic and environmental factors such as sun exposure, smoking and use of alcohol, as well as emotional stress play a role in upper facial aging.

A youthful forehead has no lines or wrinkles, and the brow in a male is at or above the bony orbital rim, whereas in a female it is usually arched with highest convexity at the junction of the medial two-thirds to the lateral one-third of the brow. This line usually coincides with the lateral border of the limbus.

With aging and loss of volume in the brow and periorbital region, the brows tend to descend, causing lateral hooding and flattening of the brow. This results in the appearance of a smaller eye, and many patients will complain of looking tired despite many hours of sleep and rest. In addition, these patients often have horizontal wrinkles on the forehead from subconsciously repeatedly raising their brows.

Some patients are very expressive in their face and with continual flexing of the corrugator and procerus muscles in the forehead, the patients can develop glabellar frown lines that are deep and visible even without flexing.

The brows and upper eyelids are interrelated, and changes in 1 area affect the other. With age, the brow fat attenuates and leads to loss of support and tissue descent that can also lead to lateral hooding and enhance upper eyelids' skin redundancy. In addition, loss of volume in the periorbital area and weakening of the orbital septum and laxity of the orbicularis-retaining ligaments produce aged contours, hollowing of the upper eyelid, and skin redundancy. Repeated flexing of orbicularis muscle and cutaneous aging results in lateral canthal lines or crow's feet, which also contribute to upper facial aging.

Laxity of the lower eyelid and fat protrusion can result in increased scleral show and lateral canthal rounding and give the patient a tired and aged appearance. In addition, the descent of the malar fat pad and exposure of the inferior orbital rim accentuate the nasojugal groove or the tear trough deformity.

Surgical technique

In the last 2 decades, volume loss has been recognized to be a major factor in upper facial aging, and thus the use of fillers has increased exponentially on a yearly basis. There are a slew of fillers available in the market, and new ones are in the pipeline; the ideal filler is yet to be found, however.

Fillers can be classified into several categories:

1. Autologous fillers (fat, cartilage, dermis, fascia, collagen from patient's skin)

[a] Inland Cosmetic Surgery, 8680 Monroe Ct, Rancho Cucamonga, CA 91730, USA
[b] Southern California Center for Surgical Arts, 4910 Van Nuys Boulevard, Suite 102, Sherman Oaks, CA 91403, USA
* Corresponding author.
E-mail address: Jhaiavy@yahoo.com

Atlas Oral Maxillofacial Surg Clin N Am 24 (2016) 105-116
1061-3315/16/$ - see front matter © 2016 Elsevier Inc. All rights reserved.
http://dx.doi.org/10.1016/j.cxom.2016.05.004

2. Biologic fillers (animal- or human-derived collagen, animal- or human-derived hyaluronic acid)
3. Synthetic fillers (Radiesse, sculptra, bellafill, Silikone 1000)

The most common fillers used in the US market are the hyaluronic acids. Hyaluronic acid is a naturally occurring hydrophilic polysaccharide found in all living cells. These materials are manufactured by recombinant technology through bacterial fermentation. The biggest advantage of the hyaluronic acid fillers is that they are hydrophilic, and they are easily reversible with an injection of an enzyme called hyaluronidase.

This is extremely important when injecting in difficult areas with thin skin such as the tear trough. In this area, too superficial an injection can result in a bluish hue under thin skin, known as the Tyndall effect. On the other hand, too much volume can result in lumpiness and exacerbation of bags under the eyes, especially when the patient is smiling.

Glabellar folds

Dynamic glabellar lines are best treated with botulinum toxins. Some glabellar folds, however, may have a deeper etched component that is best treated with filler, and therefore a combination treatment will be preferable. Oftentimes in this area, a combination of botulinum toxin and hyaluronic acid filler is used. Although both materials can be injected during the same session, it is more desirable to inject the toxin first and have the patient come back 2 weeks later for an accurate filler injection. The authors have used both Restylane and Juvederm in this location. If the lines are superficial, the material can be diluted with saline in a 1:1 ratio. A small amount of material is needed and may need to be layered in the mid-dermis to superficial dermis with a linear threading technique. When injecting superficially, temporary blanching may occur, which should be differentiated from an occlusive blanching due to intravascular injection (Figs. 1 and 2).

Forehead lines

Forehead lines are transverse lines formed by the action of the frontalis muscle in elevating the brow. Patients with dynamic forehead lines are best treated with neurotoxins. In patients with moderate-to-severe ptosis, however, caution should be exercised, as with relaxation of the frontalis, the forehead and brow ptosis worsens. For patients with deep static lines on the forehead, injection of filler may be a good option. Restylane or Juvederm can be injected to the forehead lines. If the person is thin in this area, the material can be diluted in a 1:1 ratio with saline (see Figs. 1 and 2).

Lateral canthal lines: (crow's feet)

The lateral canthal lines are formed by action of the orbiculatis oculi muscle and are influenced by sun damage and smoking. Because in most cases, these are dynamic lines, they are best treated with neurotoxins. In cases where the lines are etched in to the skin and are visible without any muscle action, an addition of filler may be indicated. In these cases, the authors use Juvederm Ultra hydrated with saline 1:1 or Restylane Silk. They use a 32 gauge needle and small amounts of material in this area; 0.2 cc or less per side.

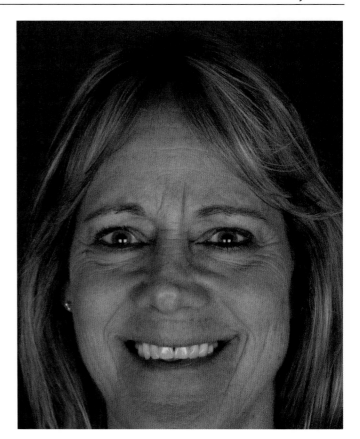

Fig. 1   Preoperative photo.

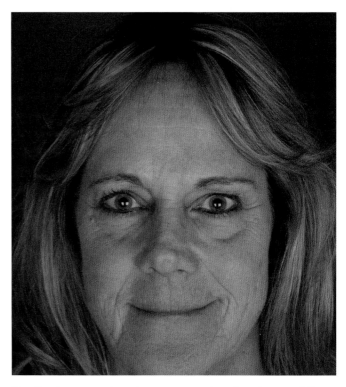

Fig. 2   Postoperative photo, status after Restylane and Botox injection to the upper face.

Periorbital, tear trough, nasojugal groove

Care should be taken when injecting fillers in the periorbital area due to thin skin and risk of retinal artery occlusion due to intravascular injection. Ideal material for filler for supraorbital and infraorbital is Belotero due to thin consistency and easy lateral spread. Lower hydrophilic properties reduce risk of both prolonged edema and Tyndell effect; Restylane silk is also a good option when injected deeper and has better property of lifting and support. Juvederm tends to produce the most edema in this area, due to large particle size and higher cross-linking, and it should be avoided unless diluted and injected submuscularly or subperiosteally. The authors use a blunt 32 gauge cannulae for injection in this area, delivering small amounts in retrograde fashion, molding to achieve the desired effect.

Temporal wasting hollowing

Sculptra can be used in the area to induce subclinical inflammatory reaction and collagen formation; the material is injected subdermally in radial fanning fashion.

Surgical technique of fat transfer

Fat is one of the oldest fillers that is biocompatible and most natural for facial rejuvenation. In the last decade, autologous fat grafting has grown in popularity, due to better understanding of the aging process as well as advancement in techniques of harvesting and transplantation of the fat cells. For patients who have significant volume loss and require global volume replacement, fat is a more ideal choice of filler (Fig. 3).

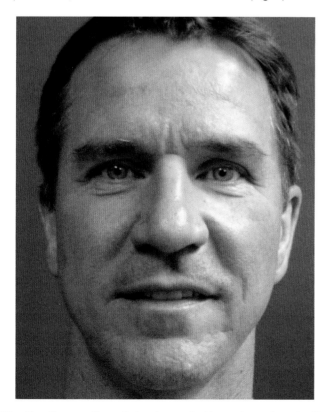

Fig. 3 Preoperative photo demonstrating volume loss in the glabella, temporal region, midface, periorbital region as well as nasolabial folds and perioral region.

Preoperative planning

Just like any cosmetic surgery patient, one who presents as a candidate for fat transfer should be evaluated with a complete history and physical examination. The surgeon must understand the patient's complaint about his or her facial appearance and evaluate the entire face, upper, middle, and lower face.

It is important to know the history of previous treatments such as injection of other fillers, botulinum toxin, or previous surgeries such as brow lift, blepharoplasty, facelifts, or previous placement of any facial implants. If the patient can provide pictures of his or her face when younger, it will help the surgeon appreciate the degree of augmentation needed.

During the physical examination, the upper face, forehead, glabella, brow, and orbits need to be evaluated with visual inspection in animation and repose as well as with palpation to get a good sense of the volume loss as well as asymmetries that are inherent to the face and skeleton. Standard photographs have to be taken and compared with previous photographs if available.

The surgeon needs to explain the procedure, recovery, possible risks, and complications to the patient. Because fat transfer is a surgical procedure, the patient needs to be ready for the down time, swelling, and bruising. In addition, options of anesthesia need to be discussed. Fat transfer can be performed under local anesthesia, although most patients in the authors' practice prefer intravenous sedation or general anesthesia, especially when combined with other procedures. The authors make a point of explaining to every patient that not all the fat transplanted survives and that they may need multiple fat transfer sessions to achieve the desired results (Fig. 4).

Preparation and patient positioning

The fat transfer procedure is usually performed under sterile conditions in an accredited surgical suite or an ambulatory surgical center. The patient is usually supine unless other areas

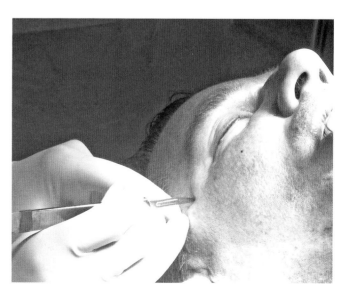

Fig. 4 Stab incision with number 11 blade for fat injection.

of liposuction are planned. Standard preparation with chlorheixidine is used over the donor site. The face is usually prepared with Benzyl Alkonium solution. The patient is draped in the standard fashion.

The donor site most commonly used is the abdomen and medial thighs, as they are easily accessible and have adequate fat reserves. If those areas are depleted due to previous liposuction or low body fat reserves, then the flanks can be another source of donor fat.

Surgical approach

Incisions for harvesting and transplantation are small (< 5 mm) and are placed in natural creases, previous scars or hair-bearing areas. For the lower abdomen and inner thighs, the incisions can be in the pubic area. For the upper abdomen, an additional incision is made in the umbilicus. For the flank area, the patient is either placed in the lateral decubitus position or the prone position. An incision is made in the lateral hip or sacral area within the panty line.

Incisions for transplantation are made in the natural creases of the forehead, glabella, or crow's feet region. For the lower eyelid and nasojugal grooves, an incision is also made in the midcheek area.

Surgical procedure

Step 1: Injection of local anesthetic

The donor site is injected with a dilute local anesthetic solution or tumescent fluid. If the patient is awake first a small wheal of 1% lidocaine with epinephrine 1:100,000 is injected at the site of insertion of cannula. A 3 mm incision is made with an 11 blade. Then the tumescent fluid (Table 1) is infiltrated in to the donor site with blunt tip multiport infiltration cannula. The tumescent fluid provides anesthesia and vasoconstriction and minimizes bleeding.

Step 2: Lipoharvesting

Harvesting can be performed with syringes (Figs. 5 and 6) or a harvesting system such as the infrasonic nutational liposuction cannula of the Tickle liposuction system (Fig. 7). In the authors' practice, 20 cc syringes with blunt tip multiport cannula (Figs. 8 and 9A) or the two-hole blunt tip Coleman cannula (Figs. 9B and 10) are used. Care is taken to minimize trauma to the fat cells harvested. The plunger of the syringe is manually drawn back only 1 mL at a time and moved gently through the fatty tissue until full. The syringe is then capped, and initially gravity is used to separate the fat cell supernatant from the serosanguinous fluid infranatant (Figs. 9C and 11). The infranatant is then discarded (Figs. 12–14).

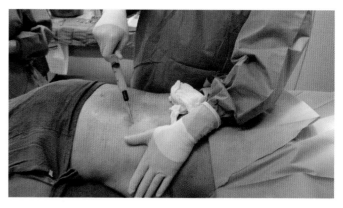

Fig. 5   Fat harvesting using syringe.

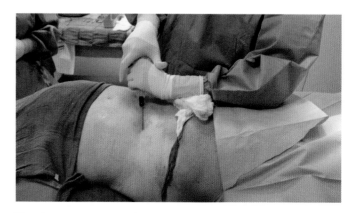

Fig. 6   Harvesting of fat with 10 cc syringes and Tulip cannula with slight negative pressure produced by hand only.

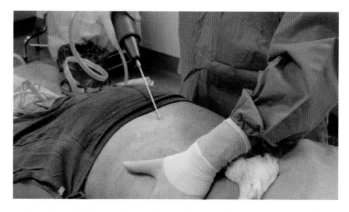

Fig. 7   Fat harvesting using Infrasonic liposuction cannula.

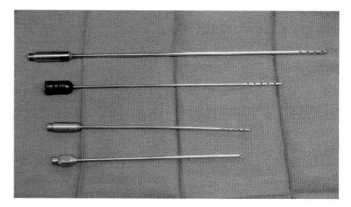

Fig. 8   Fat harvesting multiport cannulae.

Table 1   Contents of tumescent fluid

500 cc	Normal saline
25 cc	2% Lidocaine (500 mg)
1 cc	1:1000 Epinephrine

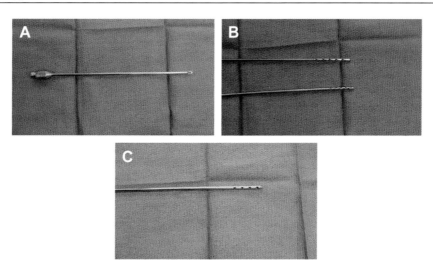

Fig. 9   (A–C) Fat harvesting cannulae.

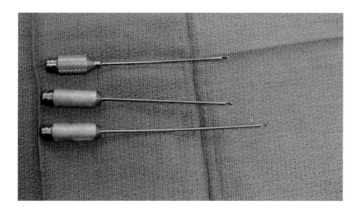

Fig. 10   Fat harvesting 2-hole cannulae.

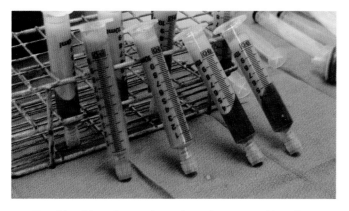

Fig. 11   Lipoasiprate decanting prior to centrifugation.

Step 3: Centrifugation and separation of components

The fat is transferred in to 10 cc syringes without the plunger and placed into a centrifuge. The syringes are then centrifuged at 3000 rpm for 3 minutes (Fig. 15). The centrifugation separates the syringe in to 3 components:

1. Top layer: least dense layer is oil from the ruptured fat cells
2. Middle layer: viable fat cells for grafting
3. Lowest level: most dense layer made up of blood, water and lidocaine

The oil is decanted first, and then the lower level fluid is allowed to flow out by removing the Luer-Lock connection (Fig. 16). Neuro-sponges (Figs. 17–19) are used to remove the rest of the oily component. It may be necessary to repeat this process a few times. The remaining fat is then transferred to 1 cc syringes for facial injections (Fig. 20).

Step 4: Injection technique

The injection is performed with blunt tip cannulas that are 0.9 mm to 1.6 mm and fit onto Luer-Lok 1 cc syringes (Fig. 21). Regional blocks such as a supraorbital nerve block, infraorbital nerve block, and zygomaticofacial and zygomaticotemporal nerve blocks are used to anesthetize the upper face. The tip of a number 11 blade is used to make an incision in a crease or a fold. The injection cannula is inserted through the incision and advanced through the tissue while the other hand stabilizes the skin. Depending on the anatomic site being injected, the fat

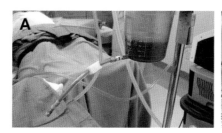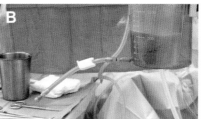

Fig. 12   (A, B) Cannister containing fat after removal of tumescent fluid and blood using attached drain.

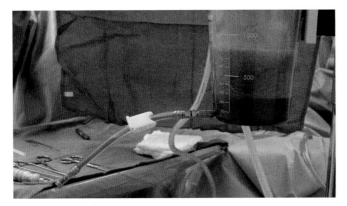

Fig. 13 Lipoaspirate in cannister prior to fluid separation and decanting.

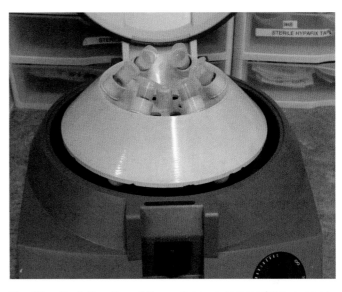

Fig. 15 Centrifugation of the syringes containing fat to separate tumescent fluid, oil and condense fat cells.

can be placed in to the subcutaneous tissues, the muscle, or above the periosteum.

The key to successful fat transplantation is atraumatic placement of the fat cells in host tissue in a manner that maximizes surface area contact and potential blood supply. The fat is injected in a retrograde fashion with multiple passes to deposit tiny amounts of fat cells in recipient tissue at different levels. The fat should be deposited carefully with the 3- dimensional anatomy and desired look in mind.

In the glabellar frown lines region, an incision is made at the superior portion of the crease. 0.9 mm Tulip cannula is used to place the fat cells in the superficial and deep subcutaneous level. Care should be taken not to inject too deep in this area due to the rich vascularity and close proximity to the orbit (Video 1).

Fat can also be deposited in the brow specifically the lateral two-thirds of the brow and in the infrabrow region. This elevates the tail of the brow and creates fullness in the brow and upper lid region, which creates a youthful anatomy (Video 2).

In the periorbital region, fat can be deposited along the lateral orbit (Video 3) and infraorbital region and the nasojugal grooves (Video 4). In the infraorbital region, the skin is thin, and the fat has to be deposited deeper in to the muscle or supraperiosteal plane to avoid visible irregularities.

Fat can also be deposited in the temporal region for older patients or postsurgical patients with temporal wasting (see Video 2).

Once the fat transplantation is complete, the incisions are closed with $1/4$ inch steristrips. There is no need for suture placement (Fig. 22).

Immediate postoperative care

Postoperatively, the patient is instructed to sleep with head of the bed elevated 30 to 40° for the following 3 nights. Ice is applied 15 minutes on and off while patient is awake for the first 24 hours to minimize swelling and bruising. The patient is reminded to keep the face clean and avoid sun exposure, heavy activity, or exercise for 3 weeks.

Potential complications

The most common adverse events with fat transfer are bruising, bleeding and rarely hematoma formation. Bruising usually resolves spontaneously with in 7 to 10 days. There is also a risk of fat necrosis, cyst formation, and calcifications.

The fat may not resorb in a uniform fashion and may lead to asymmetries that will require additional grafting for correction.

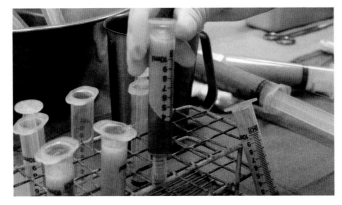

Fig. 14 Fat harvested using syringe placed to be decanted to remove tumescent fluid and blood.

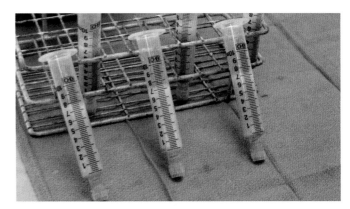

Fig. 16 Fat in syringes ready to transfer to 1 cc syringes for grafting.

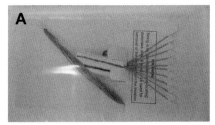
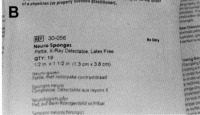

Fig. 17   (A, B) Neuro sponges used to absorb oil from centrifuged fat.

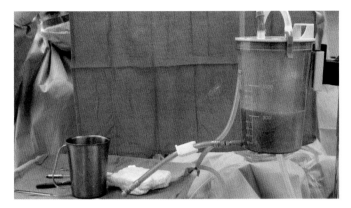

Fig. 18   Lipoaspirate prior to transfer to syringes.

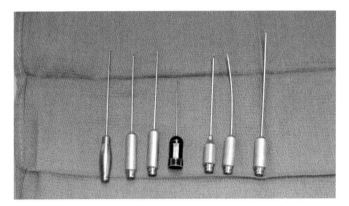

Fig. 21   Fat injection cannulae.

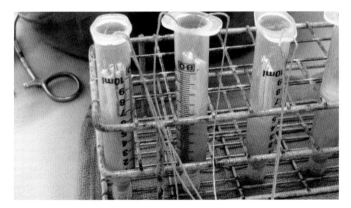

Fig. 19   Syringes containing fat after centrifugation, note neuro-sponges to absorb supernatant oil.

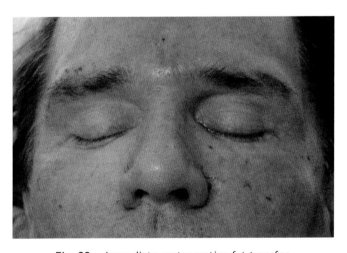

Fig. 22   Immediate postoperative fat transfer.

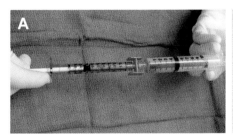
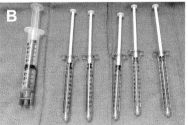

Fig. 20   (A, B) Fat transferred from 10 cc syringes to 1 cc syringes, ready for injection.

The most devastating complication is vascular occlusion. Presumably fat can be lodged in a vessel or adjacent to it, causing decreased blood flow in a given area. This becomes apparent with blanching of the skin and then a grayish blue discoloration. If insufficient collateral blood flow is present, tissue necrosis will ensue.

This complication needs immediate attention with placement of Nitropaste, massage, heat, and aspirin by mouth. If the periorbital area is being injected and patient experiences sudden pain and decreased vision, the procedure needs to be stopped and an immediate ophthalmologic evaluation obtained.

In summary, fat is a natural filler with multiple applications for facial rejuvenation. Being that it is an autologous material, it is safe, and when used properly, it provides a long-term solution to facial volume loss and laxity.

Figs. 23 and 24 show before and after photos of fat transfer.

Rehabilitation and recovery

Injectable fillers are typically done on outpatient basis with minimal to no recovery time; some degree of swelling and bruising can be expected after injection of fillers in the upper face due to tissue vascularity. Several homeopathic formulations exist to help with reducing degree of bruising and swelling after soft tissue injections such as Arnica and Bromelai. Both products can be used a 1 to 2 days prior to planned procedure and continued after the procedure for 1 to 2 days to minimize inflammatory reaction from soft tissue fillers. Patients should avoid massaging the area of injections vigorously due to risk of displacement of the soft tissue fillers. Patients should be followed for assessment of aesthetic outcome, satisfaction after procedure, and to evaluate the need for touch ups; this is usually done a week after the procedure.

Patients should be monitored for allergic reactions to fillers, granuloma formation, overcorrection or lumpiness, infections, or sterile abscess formation. Prolonged edema from hyaloronic acid (HA) fillers can result from higher crosslinked fillers with higher hydrophilic properties. Patients also should be evaluated for Tyndall effect which is bluish tint resulting from too superficial injection of the filler, common in thin skin areas such as periorbital.

Poly-L Lactic Acid (Sculptra) should be monitored for development of subcutaneous papules and nodules, which can develop weeks to months after injection. Proper dilution of the product and immediate tissue massage after injection of the product minimize the risks of nodular formation, if developed

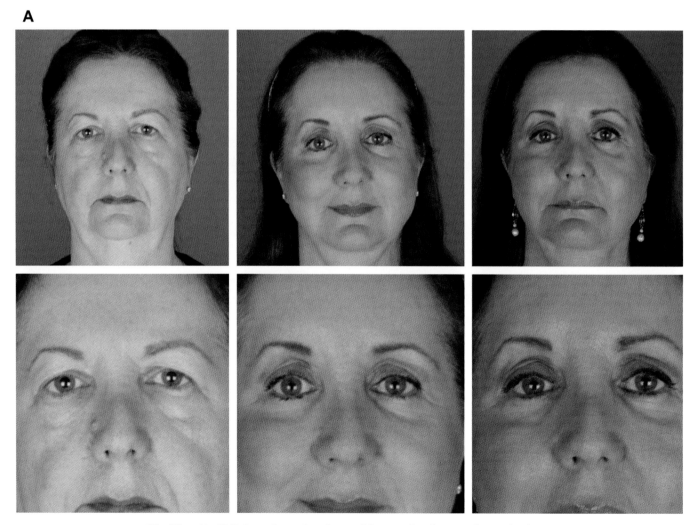

Fig. 23 *(A—C)* Before, 3 months after and 1 year after fat transfer to the face.

B

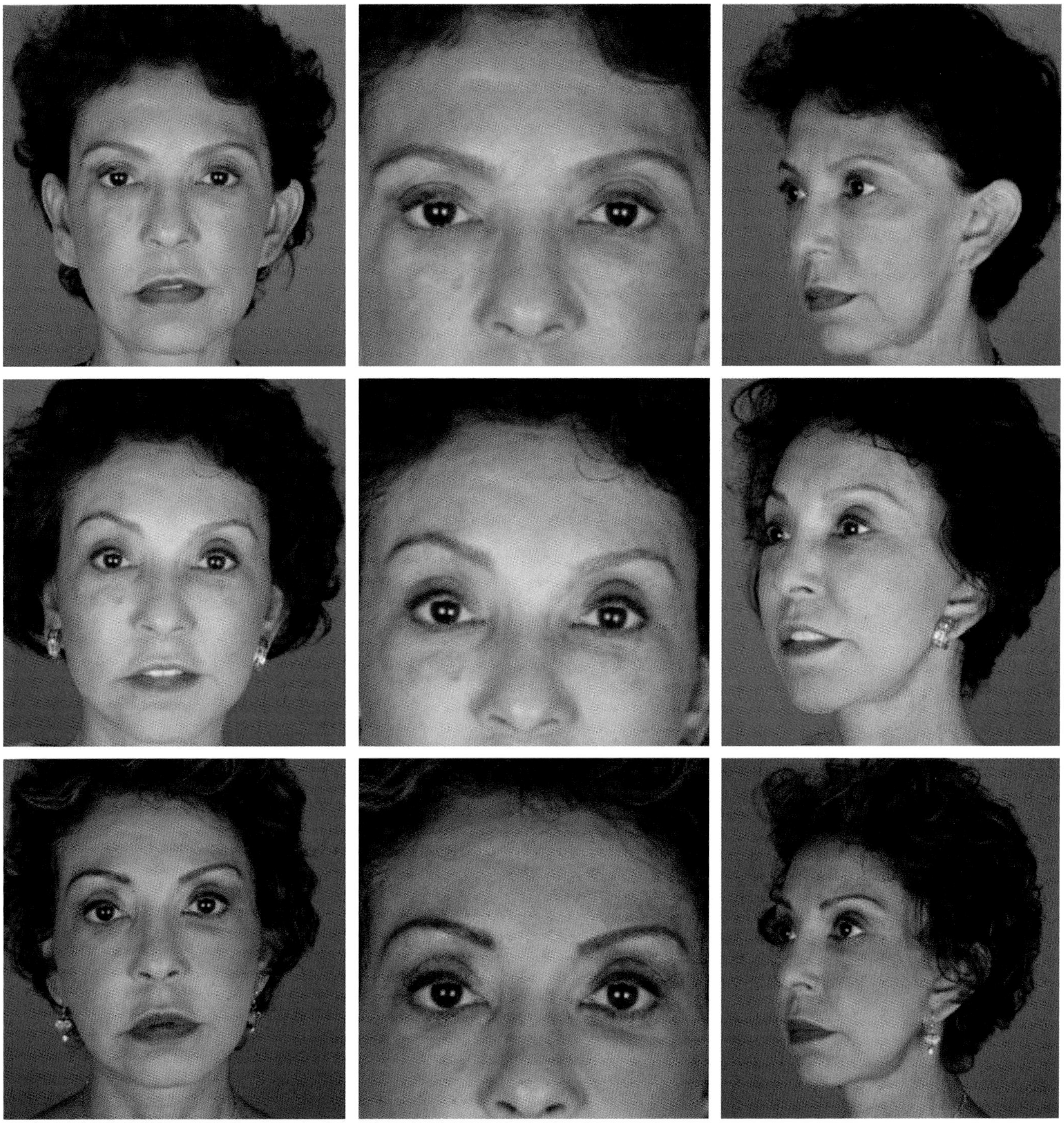

Fig. 23 *(continued)*

nodules should be managed with subcision and/or intralesional injection with steroids.

Fat transfer can result in higher degrees of swelling and bruising both to the recipient as well as the donor site. It is important to monitor donor site for hematoma or seroma formation and proper compression of the donor site to minimize dead space.

The importance cannot be overemphasized of good clinical photography before and after procedure, to monitor aesthetic clinical results, need for a touch-up and for medico-legal purposes.

Clinical results in the literature

Properties of an ideal facial filler are; biocompatible, reversible, long-lasting result, hypoallergenic or nonallergenic, inexpensive, readily available, easily acquired, non-teratogenic, and noncarcinogenic. It does not migrate after implantation, and minimal pain is associated with its acquisition and transfer. Most of currently available fillers on the market possess many of these properties; however, only autologous fat transfer satisfies most of these properties.

C

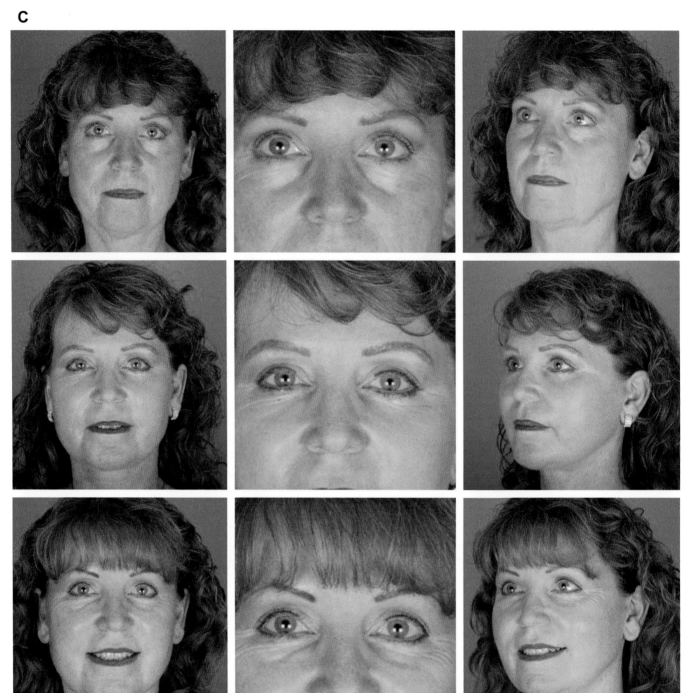

Fig. 23. (*continued*)

Hyaloronic acid soft tissue fillers

HA is a glycosaminoglycan that is a component of the extracellular matrix of the dermis. The molecule has a high water-binding capacity that plays a role in maintenance of skin moisture as well as the structure and function of the skin.

Current HA acid formulations are cross-linked nonanimal stabilized hyaluronic acids (NASHA)s derived from the fermentation of *Streptococcus equi* bacteria. The cross-linking allows for resistance to degradation by hyaloronidase in the skin. The biochemical makeup of the various HA gels (degree of cross-linking and concentration) determines their individual properties and clinical effects, such as longevity, stability, hardness, and viscosity.

Periorbital injection of fillers is considered a high-risk area due to thickness of the skin, inappropriate technique, or filler selection, which can lead to long-term fluid retention, prolonged swelling, bruising, and surface irregularities.

Restylane and Belotero HA soft tissue fillers are the most preferred in the periorbital region. Restylane has high viscosity and an elastic modulus and hence resistance to deformation and lateral spread, suitable for deep dermal injection, which allows stable fill and lift of periorbital tissue. Belotero has low

A   **B**

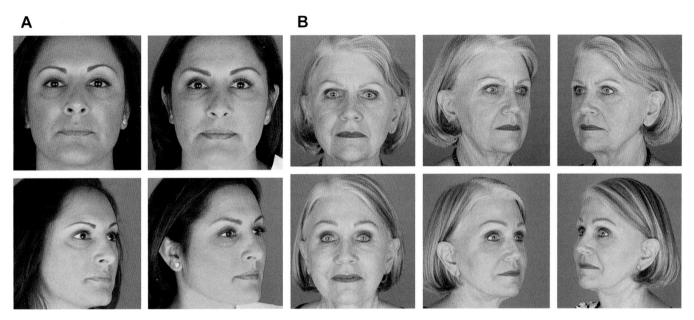

Fig. 24   (*A, B*) Before and 3 months after fat transfer to the face.

viscosity and elastic modulus and hence lower ability to fill and lift; it is suitable for use in thin skin areas with superficial injection.

Juvederm has the highest concentration of HA fillers and higher tendency to produce prolonged swelling due to hydrophilic properties; hence it reserved for glablellar and forehead lines.

Sculptra-Poly-L-Lactic acid

Poly-L-Lactic acid is a biocompatible and biodegradable synthetic polymer. Its mechanism of action is by induction of subclinical inflammatory response, which stimulates fibroblast proliferation and collagen deposition. Sculptra can be used for upper facial rejuvenation to improve lines and depression especially in the lateral brow, glabella, and temporal areas. Sculptra should be avoided in thin skin areas such as eyelids. Sculptra has been studied for use in human immunodeficiency virus (HIV)-associated lipodystrophy; several randomized trials showed efficacy in improvement of patient appearance and cutaneous thickness.

Autologous fat transfer

Lipoinjection or fat transfer has a long-lasting high success rate of achieving volumetric rejuvenation of the upper face. Fat is considered a permanent filler, hence reserved for patients who have undergone multiple treatments with temporary fillers and desire a permanent solution. Autologous fat transfer is also not recommended for the novice injector, as the results tend to be permanent and irreversible.

Controversy exists in the literature regarding the long-term survival of transplanted fat, ranging from 40% to 80% of the transplanted fat, with higher survivability with repeated injections. Improved survivability of the transplanted fat depends on several different factors: (1) atraumatic harvest of fat, (2) minimal manipulation of harvested fat, (3) smaller particles and volumes of fat injected in to deeper tissue close to muscles to enhance revascularization, and (4) careful

layering of the fat to achieve the desired effect. The choice of donor site has not been shown to be a factor in long term survival of fat.

Summary

Facial fillers remain a valuable tool in volumetric rejuvenation of the upper face alone or as an adjunct to cosmetic surgical facial procedures and neurotoxins. The injector must evaluate the need of the patient and select the appropriate filler for specific anatomic area. HA fillers are considered the workhorse of volumetric facial enhancement owing to simplicity of use, limited adverse effects, and reversibility. Autologous fat grafting is gaining more popularity with long-term predictable results. Choice of facial filler is a shared decision between the patient and the surgeon; it is important for facial surgeon to familiarize himself or herself with different types and formulation of existing facial fillers to choose the right material for the right anatomic area.

Supplementary data

Supplementary data related to this article can be found at http://dx.doi.org/10.1016/j.cxom.2016.05.004.

Further readings

Brandt FS, Cazzaniga A, Baumann L, et al. Investi- gator global evaluations of efficacy of injectable poly-L-lactic acid versus human collagen in the correction of nasolabial fold wrinkles. Aesthet Surg J 2011;31(5):521–8.

Buckingham ED. Poly-L–Lactic acid facial rejuvenation an alternative to autologous fat? Facial Plast Surg Clin North Am 2013;21(2): 271–84.

Carruthers J, Cohen SR, Joseph JH, et al. The science and art of dermal fillers for soft-tissue augmentation. J Drugs Dermatol 2009;8(4): 335–50.

Ciuci PM, Obagi S. Rejuvenation of the periorbital complex with autologous fat transfer: current ther- apy. J Oral Maxillofac Surg 2008;66(8):1686–93.

Cohen JL. Understanding, avoiding, and managing dermal filler complications. Dermatol Surg 2008;34(Suppl 1):S92—9.

Coleman SR. Facial augmentation with structural fat grafting. Clin Plast Surg 2006;33(4):567—77.

Dayan SH, Ellis DA, Moran ML. Facial fillers: discussion and debate. Facial Plast Surg Clin North Am 2012;20(3):245—64.

DeFatta RJ, Williams EF 3rd. Fat transfer in conjunction with facial rejuvenation procedures. Facial Plast Surg Clin North Am 2008; 16(4):383—90.

Ellenbogen R. Fat transfer: current use in practice. Clin Plast Surg 2000;27(4):545—56.

Eppley BL, Dadvand B. Injectable soft-tissue fillers: clinical overview. Plast Reconstr Surg 2006;118(4):98e—106e.

Glasgold RA, Glasgold MJ, Lam SM. Complications following fat transfer. Oral Maxillofacial Surg Clin N Am 2009;21(1):53—8. vi.

Hirsch RJ, Cohen JL, Carruthers JD. Successful management of an unusual presentation of impend- ing necrosis following a hyaluronic acid injection embolus and a proposed algorithm for manage- ment with hyaluronidase. Dermatol Surg 2007;33(3): 357—60.

Holck DE, Lopez MA. Periocular autologous fat transfer. Facial Plast Surg Clin North Am 2008;16(4):417—27.

Kablik J, Monheit GD, Yu L, et al. Comparative phys- ical properties of hyaluronic acid dermal fillers. Dermatol Surg 2009;35:302—12.

Lambros V. Observations on periorbital and midface aging. Plast Reconstr Surg 2007;120(5):1367—76.

Matarasso SL, Carruthers JD, Jewell ML. Consensus recommendations for soft-tissue augmentation with nonanimal stabilized hyaluronic acid (Restylane). Plast Reconstr Surg 2006;117(3 Suppl):3S—34S.

Obagi S. Specific techniques for fat transfer. Facial Plast Surg Clin North Am 2008;16(4):401—7.

Phanette G, Brown SA, Oni G, et al. Fat grafting: evidence-based re- view on autologous fat harvest- ing, processing, reinjection, and storage. Plast Reconstr Surg 2012;130(1):249—58.

Smith SR, Jones D, Thomas JA, et al. Duration of wrinkle correction following repeat treatment with Juvederm hyaluronic acid fillers. Arch Dermatol Res 2010;302(10):757—62.

Weiss RA, Weiss MA, Beasley KL, et al. Autologous cultured fibroblast injection for facial contour defor- mities: a prospective, placebo-controlled, phase III clinical trial. Dermatol Surg 2007;33(3):263—8.

Skin Resurfacing Procedures of the Upper Face

Douglas L. Johnson, DMD [a,b], Frank Paletta, MD, DMD [c,d],*

KEYWORDS

- Skin resurfacing • Fractional photothermolysis • Micro thermal zones • Fractionated CO_2 laser resurfacing

KEY POINTS

- With upper facial cosmetic surgery, the skin must be youthful appearing to give an overall esthetic appearance.
- Resurfacing has been an established treatment option for years with chemical peels and fully ablative laser treatments being the most common treatment options.
- In the appropriately selected patient, fractionated laser results are favorable and predictable for upper facial rejuvenation with limited sequelae and complications.

 Video content accompanies this article at http://www.oralmaxsurgeryatlas.theclinics.com.

Introduction

Aesthetic treatment of the upper face has been a cosmetic concern since early Egyptian times.[1] Potential changes seen in the upper facial aging are thinning or the epidermis, loss of elastic fibers and subcutaneous fat, weakening of underlying muscles, bone resorption, ptosis, and skin changes that are produced from intrinsic (chronologic) and extrinsic factors (photoaging).[2] Specific changes to the skin are seen as photo-damage: roughness, altered texture, discoloration, acral lentigines, mottled hyperpigmentation, decreased epidermal thickness, basophilic degeneration of dermis, decrease in collagen, decrease in dermal vessels, and epithelial atypia (Box 1). Upper facial rejuvenation brings with it some of the most rewarding and dramatic results for appropriately selected patients. However, in today's hyperkinetic society, many patients are demanding minimal downtime with appreciated results that compare with more traditional surgical procedures. When exploring the possibilities for skin resurfacing procedures of the upper face, there are many options a patient can be presented; each has its indications and limitations. The options range from superficial skin topical treatments with retinoids, α-hydroxy acids, and antioxidants to more ablative procedures of dermabrasion, chemical peels, and laser resurfacing.

All cosmetic lasers work by absorption of laser light to a certain selective chromophor (blood, melanin, water, etc). The gold standard for facial skin resurfacing is the carbon dioxide (CO_2; 10,600 nm)[3,4] laser. This modality can give predictably satisfying results but comes with greater risks and complications.[2] Pain, swelling, infections, prolonged recovery, hyperpigmentation or hypopigmentation, and scarring must be discussed and understood in detail. To minimize these sequelae/complications, initially nonablative technologies were explored. Rejuvenation technology of near infrared 1319 to 1320 nm, intense pulsed light, 532 nm potassium titanyl phosphate, and 585 to 595 nm pulsed dye lasers were explored, but gave minimal skin tightening affects.[4–6] This shortcoming led to the exploration of nonablative fractional photothermolysis. Fractional photothermolysis is a concept of creating microscopic thermal wounds into the skin that allows for more rapid healing.[2,6–8] The first commercial nonablative fractional photothermolysis 1550 nm was cleared by the US Food and Drug Administration for the treatment of periorbital rhytids, pigmented lesions, melasma, skin resurfacing, acne scars, and surgical scars.[5] Patients had little to no downtime and tolerated the procedures well, most of the time needing between 4 and 6 treatments. There are many devices that are available currently.

The evolution of nonablative fractional photothermolysis lasers to ablative lasers occurred to try to obtain results more resembling traditional fully ablative resurfacing. There are many wavelengths that can be used, but CO_2 and Er:YAG (2940 nm) lasers are the 2 most commonly used currently. Er:YAG lasers have a 25-fold greater affinity for water when compared with CO_2 lasers.[9] This allows the Er:YAG laser to ablate tissue well but does not produce significant lateral thermal heating, which results in less ultimate tissue tightening. The goal of this treatment is to reduce facial rhytids, skin irregularities, lentigines, keratoses, benign and precancerous lesions, reduction/removal of dyschromias or uneven pigmentations, and acne scars/scarring[3–5,7] (Box 2).

[a] Private Practice, 1301 Plantation Island Drive, Unit #101, Saint Augustine, FL 32080, USA
[b] Department of Oral & Maxillofacial Surgery, University of Florida, 655 West 8th Street, Jacksonville, FL 32209, USA
[c] Department of Surgery, Warren Alpert Medical School of Brown University, 593 Eddy Street, APC 4, Providence, RI 02903, USA
[d] Division of Oral & Maxillofacial Surgery, Department of Craniofacial Science, University of Connecticut, 263 Farmington Avenue, Farmington, CT 06030, USA
* Corresponding author. Private Practice, 243 Jefferson Boulevard, Warwick, RI 02888.
E-mail address: docpaletta@cox.net

Atlas Oral Maxillofacial Surg Clin N Am 24 (2016) 117-124
1061-3315/16/$ - see front matter © 2016 Elsevier Inc. All rights reserved.
http://dx.doi.org/10.1016/j.cxom.2016.05.010

Box 1. Aging factors

Intrinsic Aging Factors
- Epidermis thins
- Dermis and bones shrink
- Fine wrinkles
- Pigmented spots, lentigenes
- Dry skin
- Muscles weaken
- Loss of elastic fibers
- Fat on face decreases, psuedofat herniation

Extrinsic Aging Factors
- Epidermis thickens
- Dermis thins
- Coarse wrinkles, deep wrinkles, furrows
- Mottled, uneven, roughened skin
- Skin growths
- Epithelial atypia

This treatment can have minimal to moderate downtime (0–7 days typically), may require a form of topical, local, or intravenous anesthesia, and may require multiple treatments to gain the best ultimate results. This controlled skin ablation and thermal coagulation leads to improved skin texture and reduction of fine lines as well as dermal tightening and shrinkage for wrinkle reduction.[2,7] Histologic evidence of neocollagenesis is noted at 1 month, continued collagen maturation until 4 to 6 months, and may continue to evolve over 1 year to see the final tightening effect.[4]

The ablative fractionated lasers work much the same as the traditional lasers, but the beam is split by a lens into several microbeams.[7] Instead of ablating all the skin tissue, partial ablation is performed creating columns (microthermal zones) while leaving a percent of the skin intact.[10] The microcolumn healing process occurs through delivery of the degenerated necrotic tissue outward to the epidermis, known as microscopic epidermal necrotic debris, which is unique to fractional thermolysis.[5,10] The skin healing process from the pilosebaceous unit, serving as the progenitors from their base up the hair shaft and then out laterally is also known as *epiboly*.[3] This type of ablation allows for fewer overall complications, especially quicker recovery, less erythema, and decreased risk of pigmentation changes or scarring with high patient satisfaction (Box 3). Depending on the parameters used, multiple treatments many be indicated to gain the ultimate desired results. Each laser system has its own protocol for treatment. The fractionated laser pulse usually can be selected to a variable scanning size and shape to assist in treating different topographic areas of the face. The parameters may also allow the operator to

Box 2. Goals of fractionated laser resurfacing

- Reduce rhytids.
- Reduce skin irregularities.
- Reduce lentigines, keratosis, and benign precancerous lesions.
- Reduce dyschromias or uneven pigmentations.
- Reduce acne scarring or scars.

Box 3. Benefits of fractionated laser treatment

- Fewer overall complications
- Quicker recovery
- Less erythema
- Decreased risk of pigmentation changes or scarring
- High patient satisfaction

select how the pattern is delivered to the skin (Videos 1–3). These computer pattern generated (linear lines, zig zag lines, random, etc) injuries spread the heat in the tissue and may help with comfort. Specific settings of the laser beam may include output power (Watts) that determine the depth of penetration; percent of coverage, determined by the distance between each column in the treated region; and the length of time the laser beam column stays in contact with the surrounding tissues (dwell time), this determines the amount of collateral tissue injury. The zone of surrounding residual thermal damage is more important in neocollagenesis than the depth of ablation.[4] But, there is some thought that ablative fractionated lasers may be superior to traditional resurfacing devices for skin tightening in that they can penetrate deeper into the dermis with lower risks of adverse events.[8] The current fractionated laser the author uses also allows for a pulsed emission that consists of a rapid ablation of the epidermis and the first layers of the derma, whereas the second part of the pulse has low peak power allowing for targeted heating of the deeper areas of the skin.[11] Although these are individual settings, they all interplay with each other and are dependent on the condition(s) being treated and the patient's desires, resulting in a variety of results. As the parameters are escalated to obtain more dramatic results, the length of recovery and risks increase proportionately.

Before any ablative skin resurfacing procedure is performed, a standard thorough workup is indicated. Contraindications to laser skin resurfacing may include history of hypertrophic scarring/keloid formation, systemic isotretinoin within 1 year, previous recent medium to aggressive resurfacing procedure, recent open flap procedures within 6 months, immunocompromised patients, autoimmune and collagen vascular diseases, severe herpetic outbreaks, and pregnancy/current lactation.[3,4] Diseases such as vitiligo and psoriasis, which have koebnerizing features, are considered relative contraindications[6] (Box 4). Once the patient is deemed an appropriate candidate, each practitioner will have their own specific algorithm from skin

Box 4. Contraindications to laser skin resurfacing

- History of hypertrophic scarring/keloid formation
- Systemic isotretinoin (within 6–12 months)
- Recent medium to aggressive resurfacing procedure
- Recent open flap cosmetic procedure
- Severe herpetic outbreaks
- Collagen vascular diseases
- Pregnancy/current lactation

Relative contraindications
- Vitiligo, psoriasis, koeberizing features
- Immunocompromised patients

preparation to postoperative care. Depending on the patient's skin classification (Fitzpatrick, Glogau, Baumann, etc) the practitioner may recommend certain topical products. There are too many products to discuss in detail in this article, but may include a cleaner, toner, topical retinoid/tazarotene, bleaching agents (hydroquinone/kojic acid/azelaic acid), and sun blocks. Antioxidants such as vitamins E and C are common agents to combat oxygen radicals and appeal to the public as wholesome, natural substances.[12] Microdermabrasion and light chemical peels may also help to prepare the skin for a more predictable resurfacing procedure. Some of these products may be stopped a few days before the procedure to decrease sensitivity of the procedure.

Alternative options are discussed with the patient in detail. Medical microneedling is an entry-level skin resurfacing procedure. There are many proprietary devices that create small channels in the skin to standard or programmed depths. There is no thermal effect, but the microchannels can create new collagen and elastin stimulation, known also as collagen induction therapy. Certain products can be placed topically to help potentially aid in skin maturation and healing. Dermabrasion, although still practiced by some, has fallen out of mainstream favor for newer technologies mainly owing to it being technique sensitive and potentially hazardous with blood borne pathogens. Chemical peels remain a mainstay in skin resurfacing. Chemical peels come in a variety of types. Chemical peels have a mechanism of action that determine their effect and efficacy as well as different concentrations that also affect their performance. Concentration percentage is a common way to categorized peels and should be formulated by a reputable pharmacy. Trichloroacetic acid peels are common and can be applied to a level that gives predictable results. Depending on the patient's desires, a light peel can be performed, having minimal downtime and risks. These peels can be performed in a series, 1 approximately every 2 weeks for 3 to 5 treatments. A medium peel can increase the results but brings with it more downtime and risks. A medium peel can also be incorporated with a pretreatment (eg, Jessners solution) to help produce enhanced results without the risks of multiple coats. Deep phenol peels can be performed by those with judicious experience. They must be performed in smaller regional units under cardiac monitoring.

Surgical technique

Once a patient has been deemed an appropriate candidate for a fractionated laser treatment (Fig. 1), certain ancillary topics must be addressed. If the patient has had oral/facial herpes outbreaks in the past, the risk with this in the perilaser timeframe must be discussed and appropriate antiviral coverage if indicated (acyclovir, valacyclovir, famciclovir). Antibiotic coverage is a controversial topic that has no set standard, but per treating doctor may be indicated. Steroids may be administered before and after treatment. Determining the type of anesthesia for the treatment usually depends on patients' subjective pain tolerance, depth of treatment, extent of adjunctive cooling devices (forced cooling device, {SynerCool}, or a hand held fan; Fig. 2) and the ability to perform intravenous or general anesthesia.

If a light to medium resurfacing procedure is being performed, the patient presents 1 hour before treatment. An oral analgesic (hydrocodone/acetaminophen) and valium are administered as well as topical anesthetic (lidocaine/eutectic mixture of local anesthetics; Fig. 3). The patient

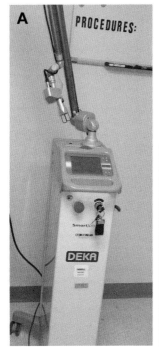
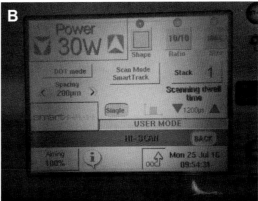

Fig. 1 (*A*, *B*) Fractionated laser treatment equipment. (DEKA, Calenzano, Italy.)

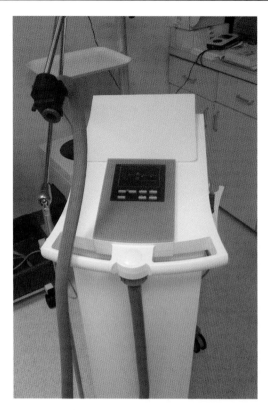

Fig. 2 Adjunctive cooling device.

also takes an oral antibiotic (Keflex 500 mg if no contraindications). The patients would have started an antiviral (acyclovir 400 mg 3 times a day) the day before the treatment. The surgical suite follows laser safety precautions. If intravenous anesthesia is being performed, appropriate monitors are in place and supplemental oxygen is turned off

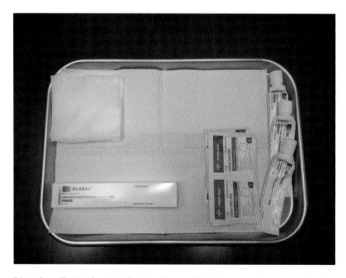

Fig. 3 Topical anesthetic for a light to medium resurfacing procedure. (Global Pharmaceuticals, Hayward, CA.)

while the laser treatment is being directly performed. The topical anesthetic is wiped off completely; the skin is cleaned with a cleanser and degreased with acetone, and then rewiped with sterile water and dried thoroughly. External laser safety eyeshields or, if periorbital resurfacing is being performed metal corneal shields, are used. Topical anesthetic eye drops (tetracaine 0.5% ophthalmic solution) then the corneal shields with lubricant (Lacralube or ophthalmic antibiotic ointment) are placed. Moistened towels are placed around the periphery of the face to aid in fire safety. Use of a smoke evacuator to remove the plume is recommended. Test spots are performed usually near the forehead to evaluate skin response and patient tolerance. At this point, units are treated without overlapping to prevent overtreatment and grid marking/stacking lines. Certain units must be treated less aggressively—over the cheek bones, periorbitally, and along the jaw line to minimize untoward potential of ectropion or scaring. For deeper rhytids and furrows, the skin should be stretched under tension and higher energy with longer dwell times used and multiple passes may be indicated. Feathering at the periphery to blend the affect is suggested. Depending on the desired results, a second pass may be indicated in deeper furrows/lines or a full second pass may be used. The char may be wiped off between passes and left after the last pass to act as a wound dressing. Fine pinpoint bleeding may be encountered and is common if at the reticular dermis level. Once the treatment is complete, iced saline soaked 4 × 4s are placed serially and changed to cool the skin and aid in comfort. An emollient (Aquaphor, or any proprietary cream that one desires to prescribe) is placed judiciously before discharge.

Rehabilitation and recovery

Patients are given posttreatment instructions at their prelaser consult. All supplies are suggested to be obtained pretreatment through a standard postprocedure care kit or over-the-counter products if acceptable substitutes. Immediately after the procedure upon arriving home, it is suggested the patient rest with their head elevated. Continued 4 × 4 or towel ice soaks can be used for comfort. It is important for the patient to keep a clean environment and wash their hands before and after caring for the area. Every 3 to 4 hours, the patient is instructed to use 0.25% acetic acid (1 tablespoon white vinegar and 1 pint warm water) or a nonmentholated shaving cream to clean the treated surface areas (this makes application easy for the patient to visualize) massaging lightly with their fingertips. The area is gently rinsed with warm water. After patting dry with a clean towel, the patient coats the resurfaced area with a light film of recovery cream/emollient. The patient is instructed they can shower and bathe normally, avoiding having shampoo or hot water running onto the treated sight. Mild to moderate redness is expected for 7 to 10 days if moderate to deep laser treatment is performed. Erythema can persist for 1 to 4 months. It is a result of induced inflammatory response, reduced melanin absorption of light, and reduced optical scattering.[6] Mild to moderate swelling is normal for 3 to 7 days; if periorbital treatment is performed, the eyes may swell and visual fields decreased for 2 to 4 days. Oozing of clear fluid or "weeping" from the resurfaced sites may occur for 1 to 3 days. Helping to removed scabs by scaling or picking should be avoided and may leave a scar or cause hyperpigmentation. The patient is reminded the skin is in a delicate transition stage and must be treated gently. All prescription medication is taken as directed. Pruritus, which is not uncommon and usually self-limited, can be treated with an over-the-counter antihistamine and mild topical steroid if indicated. The patient is instructed to avoid direct sun exposure for at least 3 months. Makeup and sunscreen may be applied after the skin has rejuvenated; bland, nonscented, PABA-free products are recommended. Routine daily activities can begin at 7 to 10 days, and routine skin care products can usually be restarted at about the third week. The patient is reminded it

Box 5. Fractionated laser posttreatment sequelae/complications

- Erythema/edema
- Hyperpigmentation/hypopigmentation
- Infection (bacterial, viral, fungal)
- Pruritus
- Contact dermatitis
- Milia
- Acne
- Scarring

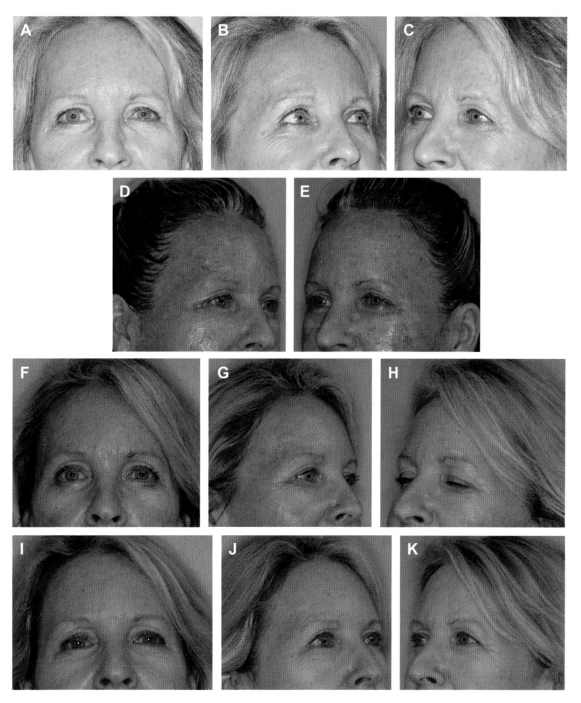

Fig. 4 Case 1 (see corresponding Video 1). (*A*) Before laser treatment, frontal. (*B*) Before laser treatment, right. (*C*) Before laser treatment, left. (*D*) After laser treatment, day 3, right. (*E*) After laser treatment, day 3, left. (*F*) After laser treatment, day 7, frontal. (*G*) After laser treatment, day 7, right. (*H*) After laser treatment, day 7, left. (*I*) Final result after laser treatment, frontal. (*J*) Final result after laser treatment, right. (*K*) Final result after laser treatment, left.

Johnson & Paletta

will take 4 to 6 months to potentially see the final tightening affects.

The safety profile for fractionated lasers is excellent when the units are used appropriately. Most patients resume normal work/social activities within 7 to 10 days.[13] Posttreatment sequelae and adverse events are much the same as with fully ablative procedures, but to a lesser extent[14] (Box 5). Erythema, as mentioned, is typically of short duration and easily managed. Ruling out contact sensitivity is important, and infrequently topical steroids can be used. Depigmentation is a result of the depth of treatment. Postinflammatory hyperpigmentation is the most common adverse effect of laser treatment,[6] especially in the darker tone skin types. It is seen less with fractionated laser treatment and is usually responsive to pharmacologic treatment (hydroquinone and tretinoin) and sun avoidance. True hypopigmentation is limited, even with darker skin tones.[9,13] Infections (bacterial, viral, fungal) should be mindful any time a resurfacing procedure is

performed, and appropriate workup and treatment are indicated as soon as suspected to try to minimize untoward results. Milia are usually self-declaring, but may need to be treated (unroofing, topical retinoids restarted, diathermy, curettage, cryotherapy). Contact dermatitis may occur and the offending agent should be identified and discarded. Mild antiitch lotions or mild steroid creams may be indicated. Acne flares may occur as the oil glands recover with resurfacing or may indicate too heavy of an emollient is being placed. After appropriate education, if acne persists antibiotics may be indicated topically (erythromycin or clindamycin) or systemically (decline). Scarring is a late complication with fractionated lasers, but if it does occur, must be identified and treated early. Strong topical steroids, silicone application (sheets or gel), steroid injections, and pulsed dye laser are options for treatment.

Figs. 4–6 provide preoperative and postoperative case photos.

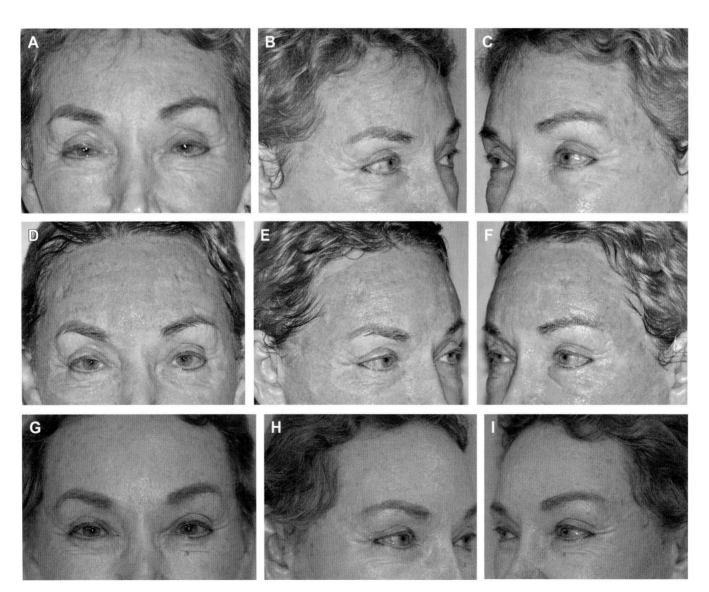

Fig. 5 Case 2 (see corresponding Video 2). (*A*) Before laser treatment, frontal. (*B*) Before laser treatment, right. (*C*) Before laser treatment, left. (*D*) After laser treatment, day 1, frontal. (*E*) After laser treatment, day 1, right. (*F*) After laser treatment, day 1, left. (*G*) After laser treatment, day 7, frontal. (*H*) After laser treatment, day 7, right. (*I*) After laser treatment, day 7, left.

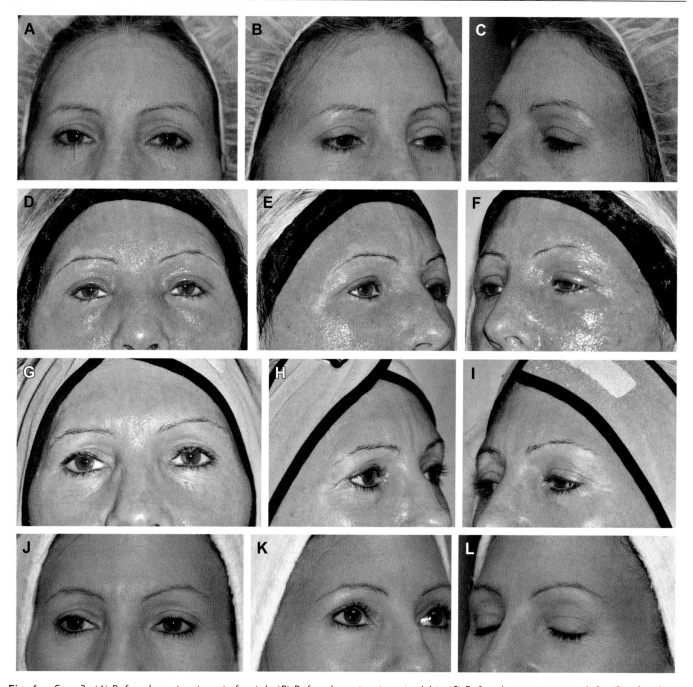

Fig. 6 Case 3. (*A*) Before laser treatment, frontal. (*B*) Before laser treatment, right. (*C*) Before laser treatment, left. (*D*) After laser treatment, day 1, frontal. (*E*) After laser treatment, day 1, right. (*F*) After laser treatment, day 1, left. (*G*) After laser treatment, day 7, frontal. (*H*) After laser treatment, day 7, right. (*I*) After laser treatment, day 7, left. (*J*) Final result after laser treatment, frontal. (*K*) Final result after laser treatment, right. (*L*) Final result after laser treatment, left.

Summary

Traditional fully ablative CO_2 laser resurfacing is an excellent treatment modality for facial rejuvenation, the results are typically well worth the risk and downtime. But in today's hyperkinetic society that is demanding to minimal downtime, minimal risks yet appreciated results, newer technologies have been advancing to try and meet these needs. Like many other technologies, there is a learning curve to and sometimes hopeful optimism that cannot meet the desires. The procedure induces skin tightening through dermal heating, wound healing, neocollagenesis and dermal remodeling. Fractionated laser CO_2 resurfacing has evolved and now can give most of the benefits of traditional resurfacing with decreasing the untoward side effects and high overall patient satisfaction.[15] The treatment can be tailored to the patient's desires allowing for versatility of treatment but ultimately obtaining overall long-term satisfying affects that have met the patients demands.

Supplementary data

Supplementary data related to this article can be found at http://dx.doi.org/10.1016/j.cxom.2016.05.010.

References

1. Beer K, Bayers S. Aesthetic treatment considerations for the eyebrows and periorbital complex. J Drugs Dermatol 2014;13(1):17–20.

2. Hunzeken C, Weiss E, Geronemus R. Fractionated CO2 laser resurfacing: our experience with more than 2000 treatments. Aesthet Surg J 2009;29:317–22.

3. Niamtu J. Skin resurfacing. In: Niamtu J, editor. Cosmetic facial surgery. St Louis (MO): Elsevier Mosby; 2011. p. 517–603.

4. Gotkin RH, Sarnoff DS, Cannarozzo G, et al. Ablative skin resurfacing with a novel microablative CO_2 laser. J Drugs Dermatol 2009; 8(2):138–44.

5. Gold M. Update on fractional laser technology. J Clin Aesthet Dermatol 2010;3(1):42–50.

6. Alexiades-Armenakas M, Dover J, Arndt K. The spectrum of laser skin resurfacing: nonablative, factional, and ablative laser resurfacing. J Am Acad Dermatol 2008;58: 719–37.

7. Tresses M, Shohat M, Urdiales F. Safe and effective one-session fractional skin resurfacing using a carbon dioxide laser device in super-pulse mode: a clinical and histologic study. Aesthetic Plast Surg 2011;35:31–42.

8. Ortiz A, Goldman M, Fitzpatrick R. Ablative CO_2 lasers for skin tightening: traditional versus fractional. Dermatol Surg 2014;40:S147–51.

9. Obagi S. Fractionated laser. SURGE, a publication of the AACS 2015;(1):20–1.

10. Lipozencic J, Makos Z. Will nonablative rejuvenation replace ablative lasers? Facts and controversies. Clin Dermatol 2013;31: 718–21.

11. Le Pillouer-Prost A. Fractional laser skin resurfacing with SmartXide DOT. Initial Results. Italy: Deka s.r.l; 2008. p. 1–4.

12. Hegedus F, Diecidue R, Taub D, et al. Non-surgical treatment modalities of facial photodamage: practical knowledge for the oral and maxillofacial professional. Int J Oral Maxillofac Surg 2006;35: 389–98.

13. Khaled M, Benedetto A. Facial skin rejuvenation: ablative laser resurfacing, chemical peels, or photodymanic therapy? Facts and controversies. Clin Dermatol 2013;31:737–40.

14. Duplechain J. Fractional CO_2 resurfacing has it replaced ablative resurfacing techniques? Facial Plast Surg Clin North Am 2013;21: 213–27.

15. Kohl E, Meirhofer J, Koller M, et al. Fractional carbon dioxide laser resurfacing of rhytids and photoaged skin- a prospective clinical study on patient expectation and satisfaction. Lasers Surg Med 2015;47:111–9.

Upper Eyelid Blepharoplasty

Michael J. Will, MD, DDS

KEYWORDS

• Upper eyelid blepharoplasty • Brow lifting procedure • Periorbital region

KEY POINTS

• Upper eyelid blepharoplasty has become more conservative, where there is less excision and more emphasis on repositioning and restoring orbital anatomy and volume.
• Thorough periorbital preoperative evaluation is necessary to determine the appropriate blepharoplasty procedure with or without the need for a brow lifting procedure.
• Conservative approaches that reduce the risk of complications such as lagophthamous should always be considered.
• Periorbital skin quality improvement and reduction of rhytids may require skin tightening or resurfacing procedures in addition to blepharoplasty as adjunctive therapy.
• Ancillary procedures such as neurotoxin or dermal filler injections may be combined with blepharoplasty techniques to provide more complete rejuvenation and a higher degree of patient satisfaction.

Introduction

The periorbital region is one of the earliest and primary locations on the face where patients seek rejuvenation. When we interact and speak to one another, we tend to look at each other's eyes for signs of approval, understanding, and any emotional responses elicited. Therefore, the patients who are considering facial rejuvenation typically begin their quest for a more youthful appearance by pursuing periorbital cosmetic procedures. Frequently, patients state during the consultation with their cosmetic surgeon that they do not like their aging face as a whole; however, they emphasize that they would like to start by rejuvenating their eyes. If the periorbital cosmetic procedures go well and result in a high degree of patient satisfaction, the patient gains confidence in cosmetic surgery and frequently goes on to rejuvenate other cosmetic regions of the face and body.

Anatomy of the periorbital region

The eyebrow position, shape, and form must be considered along with the eyelids and periorbital skin when evaluating this region for age-related changes and surgical rejuvenation. Cosmetic surgery of the brow and forehead will be discussed in other articles (see Tirbod Fattahi's article, "Open Brow Lift Surgery for Facial Rejuvenation" and Jon D. Perenack's article, "The Endoscopic Brow Lift," in this issue); however, the aging brow must be given equal attention when considering cosmetic surgery of the eyelids and surrounding skin.

The upper eyelid anatomy must be clearly understood, with each layer identified when traversing through the lid to address cosmetic concerns (Fig. 1). The Caucasian eyelids should demonstrate a dominant lid crease 8 to 11 mm from the palpebral margin, and if absent with a deep upper lid sulcus, may indicate levator disinsertion and eyelid ptosis (Figs. 2 and 3). This eyelid crease in the Caucasian patient is at 8 to 11 mm from the palpebral margin and represents a line of fusion of levator aponeurosis with the tarsal plate with its concomitant dermal attachments providing the crease (Fig. 4). In the Asian eyelid, this line of fusion is below the cephalic margin of the tarsal plate, which allows some preaponeurotic fat to extend over the tarsal plate and diminish the appearance of a tarsal crease. The skin overlying the tarsal plate, which is about 8 to 10 mm in length, is considered the pretarsal skin that overlays the pretarsal orbicularis oculi muscle. The skin superior to the tarsal plate is the preseptal skin overlying the preseptal obicularis oculi muscle (Fig. 5).[1,2]

Superior to the tarsal plate and just below the obicularis oculi muscle lays the orbital septum, which originates from the periorbita and inserts into the undersurface of the tarsal plate and fuses with the levator aponeurosis. Just deep to the orbital septum lays the preaponeurotic fat that is contained in 2 compartments, the central and medial fat pads (Fig. 6). The lateral space that would contain the lateral pad, if it existed, is occupied by the lacrimal gland. The medial fat fad is typically lighter in color than the central fat fad, and the lacrimal gland is more orange in color and more vascular on its surface. Fullness of the upper eyelid is frequently due to attenuation of the orbital septum, allowing preaponeurotic fat to bulge forward (pseudofat herniation) (see Fig. 1).[2]

Fullness of the eyelids can be related to endocrine disease and other systemic disorders that must be ruled out before performing blepharoplasty. Deep to the preaponeurotic fat lays the levator aponeurosis and the levator palpebrae superioris muscle. These structures must be preserved and respected during cosmetic eyelid surgery to prevent levator disinsertion and subsequent ptosis. This layer is addressed for ptosis repair surgery through levator suspension. The only

Will Surgical Arts, 3280 Urbana Pike, Suite 201, Ijamsville, MD 21754, USA
E-mail address: drwill@willsurgicalarts.com

Atlas Oral Maxillofacial Surg Clin N Am 24 (2016) 125–133
1061-3315/16/$ - see front matter © 2016 Elsevier Inc. All rights reserved.
http://dx.doi.org/10.1016/j.cxom.2016.05.008

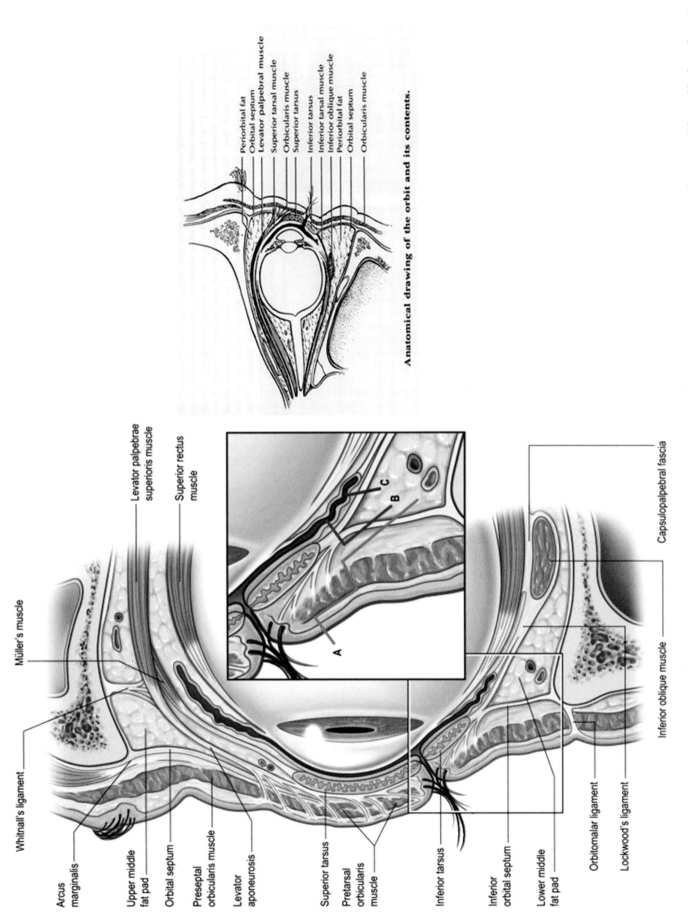

Periorbital fat
Orbital septum
Levator palpebral muscle
Superior tarsal muscle
Orbicularis muscle
Superior tarsus

Inferior tarsus
Inferior tarsal muscle
Inferior oblique muscle
Periorbital fat
Orbital septum
Orbicularis muscle

Anatomical drawing of the orbit and its contents.

Levator palpebrae superioris muscle

Superior rectus muscle

Müller's muscle

Whitnall's ligament

Arcus marginalis

Upper middle fat pad

Orbital septum

Preseptal orbicularis muscle

Levator aponeurosis

Superior tarsus

Pretarsal orbicularis muscle

Inferior tarsus

Inferior orbital septum

Lower middle fat pad

Orbitomalar ligament

Lockwood's ligament

Inferior oblique muscle

Capsulopalpebral fascia

Fig. 1   Cross-sectional anatomy of the eyelids with subciliary (A) and transconjunctival incision outine (B and C). (*From* Saadeh P. Conventional upper and lower blepharoplasty. In: Aston S, Steinbrech DS, Walden JL, editors. Aesthetic plastic surgery. St Louis (MO): Elsevier; 2012. p. 325; with permission).

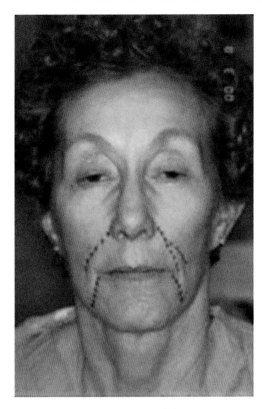

Fig. 2   Bilateral eyelid ptosis.

layer remaining before encountering the globe, once deep to the levator, is the palpebral conjunctiva. Therefore, levator suspension procedures require the use of globe protection in the way of a shield to prevent injury to the bulbar conjunctiva.

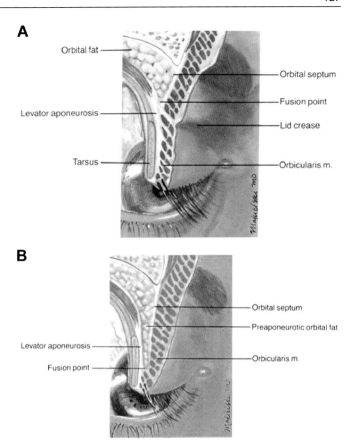

Fig. 4   Non-Asian upper eyelid anatomy (*A*); Asian eyelid anatomy (*B*). m., muscle. (*From* Larrabee WF, Makielski KH. Surgical anatomy of the face. New York: Raven Press, 1993; with permission.)

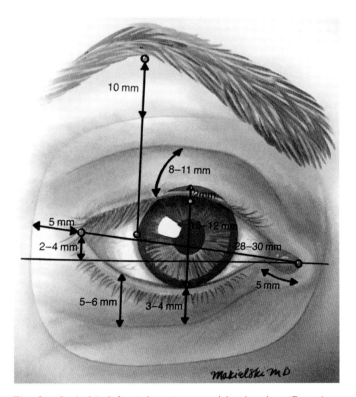

Fig. 3   Periorbital frontal anatomy and landmarks. (*From* Larrabee WF, Makielski KH. Surgical anatomy of the face. New York: Raven Press, 1993; with permission.)

Eyelid esthetics

The palpebral margin should demonstrate a superior lateral inclination or slant in the nonsyndromic patient. The medial portion of the palpebral margin is more vertical than the lateral forming the almond shape of the open eyelid margin. The superior eyelid margin should end at the superior limbus of the iris and not extent more than 2 mm into the iris. The upper eyelid crease does not extent medial to the fornix, except in Asian eyelids, where epicanthal folds exist. The lateral fornix should be the lateral extent of the upper eyelid crease; otherwise, lateral hooding and redundant eyelid or brow skin are present (see Fig. 2).[1,3]

Age-related changes of the periorbital region

Age-related changes of this regional cosmetic subunit must be understood in 3 dimensions and cannot be isolated to only the upper eyelids. Therefore, the age-related changes and preoperative assessment of the entire peri-orbital region to include the brows and upper and lower eyelids are discussed. Gravity and subdermal atrophy result in a decreased projection of the eyebrows and a tendency toward a lower brow position with loss of the brow arch in women, resulting in redundant eyelid and brow skin encroaching on the palpebral margin. Attenuation of the orbital septum allows pseudoherniation of fat of the fat pads and contributes to an

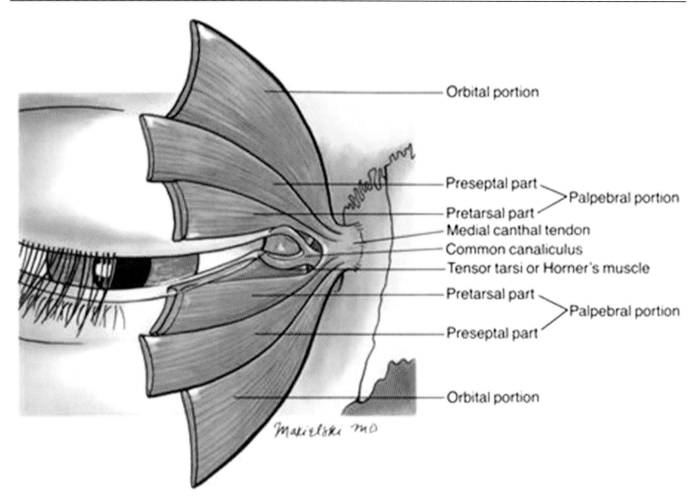

- Orbital portion
- Preseptal part ⎤
- Pretarsal part ⎦ Palpebral portion
- Medial canthal tendon
- Common canaliculus
- Tensor tarsi or Horner's muscle
- Pretarsal part ⎤
- Preseptal part ⎦ Palpebral portion
- Orbital portion

Fig. 5 Obicularis oculi muscle anatomy of the eyelids. (*From* Larrabee WF, Makielski KH. Surgical anatomy of the face. New York: Raven Press, 1993; with permission.)

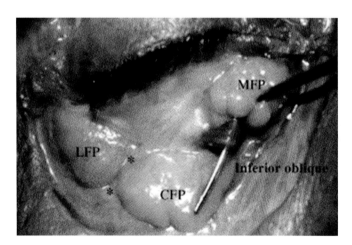

Fig. 6 Anterior view of deep dissection of right lower eyelid orbital fat pads. The inferior oblique muscle divides the medial from the central fat, and the arcuate expansion fascia (*asterisks*) of the inferior oblique muscle divides the central from the lateral fat pads. CFP, central fat pad; LFP, lateral fat pad; MFP, medial fat pad. (*From* Burkat CN, Lemke BN. Anatomy of the orbit and its related structures. Otolaryngol Clin North Am 2005;38(5):828; with permission.)

appearance of bulging or fullness of the eyelids. Dermal thinning allows discoloration of the eyelids as previously mentioned and the appearance of underlying anatomic structures, such as the orbital rim, vessels, and fat pockets. The effects of gravity and dermal and subdermal atrophy contribute to brow ptosis, dermatochalasis, periorbital rhytids, and the appearance of nasojugal folds (tear troughs) and prominent infraorbital rims. Excessive ultraviolet light and extreme environmental exposure contribute to collagen degradation and loss of elastin fibers that also result in periorbital rhytids and redundant skin. Constant squinting during extended exposure to sunny environments can lead to orbicularis hypertrophy of the lower lid pretarsal obicularis oculi muscle that may masquerade as baggy lower eyelids that may elicit cosmetic concerns from affected patients.[4]

Attenuation of the medial and lateral canthal ligaments associated with aging will result in decreased lid tone and predispose the patient to lateral canthal rounding, scleral show, ectropion, and lagophthalmos following cosmetic surgical procedures of the eyelids. A thorough understanding of these age-related changes of the periorbital region is necessary to assess and plan 3-dimensional periorbital rejuvenation using resective techniques as well as volumizing procedures where necessary.[4]

Preoperative assessment

A thorough history and physical examination are necessary to identify any systemic condition that may adversely affect the surgical outcome. A detailed ocular history is imperative, and if any significant ocular history is identified such as glaucoma, Graves disease, myasthenia gravis, visual acuity changes, or prior orbital surgery or trauma, a preoperative ophthalmology consultation is prudent. Current medications that may interfere with coagulation or platelet function should be identified and discontinued before surgical intervention if approved by the patient's primary care provider. The ocular physical examination should, at a minimum, document visual acuity, extraocular muscle function, lid tone (snap test) and function, the degree of eye lubrication, and the presence of orbital or ocular abnormality. Preoperative photographs in the frontal, oblique, and profile views in repose and smile are an absolute requirement to document the patient's baseline periorbital appearance.[4]

Assess and document the following:

- The eyelid position relative to the globe and iris
- Skin for abnormality, rhytids, thickness, redundancy, laxity, and color
- Visual presence of the infraorbital rim, nasojugal folds, malar fat pad, or cheek festoons
- Presence and position of the supratarsal fold (lid crease)
- Position and presence of the fat pads (gentle globe pressure to accentuate pseudo fat herniation)
- Eyelid excursion with opening and closing of the eyelids (check for ptosis)
- Presence of ectropion, scleral show, proptosis, enophthalmos
- Tear film management (epiphora or dry eye symptoms)
- Lid tone/tension with the lower lid distraction snap test when contemplating lower eyelid surgery
- Prominence of lacrimal gland
- Brow position identified relative to the orbital rim (brow ptosis will contribute to redundant upper lid skin). Average vertical distance from palpebral margin to the mid brow position is 27 mm[5,6]
- Patient's motivating factors and expectations as well as their impression of body image
- Thorough discussion of the risks, benefits, and alternatives as well as the limitations and expected outcomes if no complications are encountered. Delineate the most common complications and answer all questions to establish consent.

Selection of surgical procedure

The goal is to rejuvenate the periorbital structures and provide a more refreshed and youthful appearance. The regional anatomy that may need to be addressed includes the periorbital skin, muscle, lid position, and fat herniation. Skin, muscle, and fat resection of the upper eyelid is the standard approach to upper eyelid blepharoplasty; however, the same technique to address the lower eyelids frequently results in lid retraction, ectropion, scleral show, lateral canthal rounding, and a sunken appearance from excessive fat removal.[6] The trend is now toward more conservative fat removal or repositioning through a lower eyelid transconjunctival approach without violating the anterior lamellae. If there is a need for skin and/or muscle

resection, strong consideration should be given to a lower lid suspension procedure (tarsal strip) or canthopexy.[7] Skin redundancy or lid laxity may be more appropriately addressed through transconjunctival lower lid blepharoplasty with laser skin resurfacing or chemical peels to improve skin tone and tension. The choice between transcutaneous and transconjunctival blepharoplasty is dictated by the patient's anatomy, presentation, and esthetic demands. Excellent results are attainable through both techniques as long as the risk of complications is mitigated through the use of adjunctive procedures such as lower lid suspension procedures and canthopexy. Periorbital rhytids for the most part do not respond favorably to cosmetic blepharoplasty and typically require skin resurfacing, dermal fillers, and/or neurotoxins. Management of the lower eyelid and cosmetic enhancement will be covered in another article (see Gary Linkov and Allan E. Wulc's article, "Management of Lower Eyelid Laxity," in this issue).

Surgical planning and skin markings

Always mark the patients in the upright position. Traditionally, the sequence of surgery begins with surgical repositioning of the brow, followed by upper eyelid blepharoplasty and lower eyelid procedures to include skin resurfacing.

The markings for the upper eyelid begins with elevating the brow to identify the most dominant lid crease, approximately 10 mm from the palpebral margin and marked along the crease from the medial to the lateral extent of the hooding, while staying within the confines of the orbit (Fig. 7). The lateral extent may abruptly curve superiorly to eliminate hooding. The superior limb is determined by grasping lid skin superior to the lid crease and gathering the redundant tissue with a smooth forceps and increasing the vertical extent of the superior resection until lagophthalmos develops when the patients attempt to close their lids gently (Fig. 8). If medial redundancy of the skin is present, "W-plasty" modification may be necessary to prevent web formation.

Anesthesia considerations

Blepharoplasty can be safely conducted with local anesthesia alone, conscious sedation, or general anesthesia. Corneal

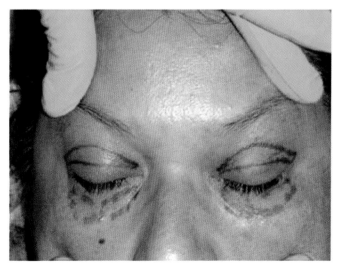

Fig. 7 Upper eyelid marking for elliptical skin excision and lower fat fad markings for transconjunctival fat excision.

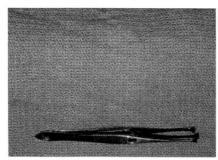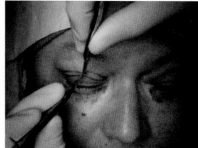

Fig. 8   Forceps to gently grasp eyelid skin to determine vertical extend of skin excision.

anesthesia can be obtained with the use of the 4% Tetracaine, and epinephrine containing local anesthetics is preferable for hemostasis. Consider intermittent corneal lubrication with balanced salt solution or Lacri-Lube during the procedure and use the corneal shields to prevent globe injuries.

Upper blepharoplasty procedure

Local anesthetic is injected into the marked areas of the upper eyelids by staying superficial and away from the globe by elevating the upper eyelid superiorly above the globe (Fig. 9). A skin muscle incision is performed along the presurgical marking lines previously described (Fig. 10). The skin muscle flap is elevated off of the septum with a needle point electrocautery or radiofrequency tip (Figs. 11 and 12). The orbital septum is then opened with an iris scissors from the lateral limbus to the medial canthal area to allow the preaponeurotic fat to herniate into the wound. Care must be taken to open the septum superiorly in the wound to stay over the preaponeurotic fat and to prevent injury to the levator system (Fig. 13). The preaponeurotic fat is grasped with fine-tip pickups and gently teased off the levator aponeurosis with a moistened cotton tip applicator. If there is an indication to reduce fullness and volume of the upper eyelids, excise central and medial fat pads conservatively. Only take what herniates through the opening of the septum. Electrocautery is necessary to amputate the herniating fat and to provide hemostasis to prevent

vessels from bleeding and retracting into the orbit (Fig. 14). The medial fat pad will require gentle globe pressure to elevate the overlying septum to allow the septum to be unroofed with a delicate scissors. This fat is lighter in color and tends to herniate in a column as teased out with grasping and separated from the surrounding tissues with a moistened cotton tip applicator. Once the desired fat is removed and the surgical field is hemostatic, a running 6-0 subcutaneous nylon or polypropylene suture is run from medial to lateral and secured with a knot or adhesive strip on either end, followed by the placement of skin adhesive strips (Figs. 15 and 16).[7–9]

Ancillary periorbital procedures

Periorbital rhytids can adjunctively be treated with laser skin resurfacing using carbon dioxide or erbium energy sources as well as the use of a medium depth chemical peel, such as trichloroacetic acid, and finally using neurotoxins and dermal fillers. Care must be taken during periorbital laser skin resurfacing to avoid excessive skin contraction and retraction that may result in ectropion, scleral show, or lateral canthal rounding. Additional potential postoperative complications include pigmentary changes, scarring, infection (viral, fungal, or bacterial), and ocular injury. Postoperative care routinely consists of moist dressings, debridement with an astringent, analgesics, antibiotics, antifungals, and antiviral medications.

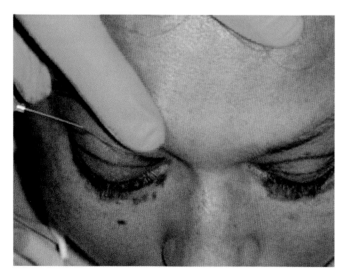

Fig. 9   Elevate the eyelid up off the globe during local anesthetic injection to prevent inadvertent globe injury.

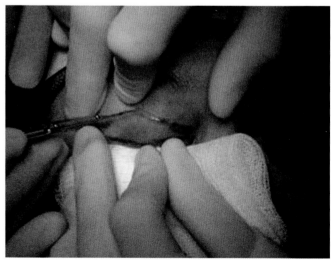

Fig. 10   Upper eyelid skin/muscle incision.

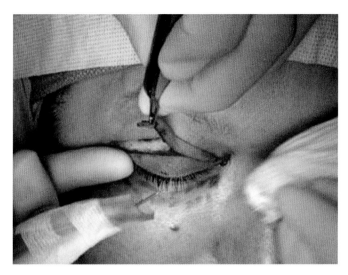

Fig. 11 Skin/muscle flap elevated and excised with needle-point electrocautery.

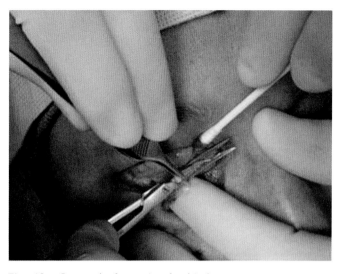

Fig. 13 Removal of a strip of orbital septum to expose pre-aponeurotic fat.

Dynamic periorbital rhytids are most effectively treated with neurotoxin injections within the lateral fibers of the orbicularis oculi muscle. Some of the infraorbital and lateral orbital dynamic rhytids with smile can be improved with neurotoxin injections within the proximal aspect of the zygomaticus major muscle over the malar process to reduce the amount of cheek rise with smile. A very low dose injection of neurotoxin (1–2 units) into the pretarsal lower eyelid orbicularis muscle can improve lower eyelid rhytids and decrease the prominence of orbicularis hypertrophy in patients who are heavy squinters.[10]

Static periorbital rhytids are best treated with the previously mentioned skin resurfacing modalities in conjunction with low viscosity dermal fillers such as the hyaluronic acid products. A detailed discussion of skin resurfacing, neurotoxin and dermal fillers are beyond the scope of this section and will be covered in other articles (see Jacob Haiavy and Husam Elias' article, "Injectable Fillers in the Upper Face" and Clement Qaqish's article, "Botulinum Toxin Use in the Upper Face," in this issue).

Postoperative care

Antibiotic ointment may be applied to the incisions or the inferior fornix following blepharoplasty. The patients are advised to avoid strenuous activity and remain in the head up position for several days postoperatively and apply ice packs during the acute phase. Moisturizing eye drops may be required to prevent dry eye symptoms during the eyelid equilibration phase postoperatively. Skin sutures are usually removed within the first week, and eyelid massage may be used for several weeks to aid in the control of edema. Ecchymosis and edema usually resolve within 2 to 3 weeks.

Complications

A thorough history and physical examination in conjunction with an accurate diagnosis and treatment plan will help set up the case for success and minimize the likelihood of postoperative complications.[11]

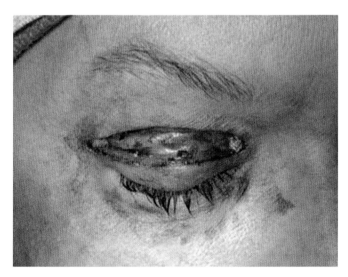

Fig. 12 Orbital septum following excision of skin/muscle flap.

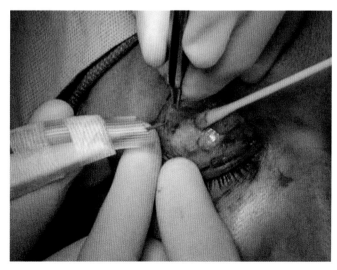

Fig. 14 Conservative removal of preaponeurotic fat, preserving the levator aponeurosis.

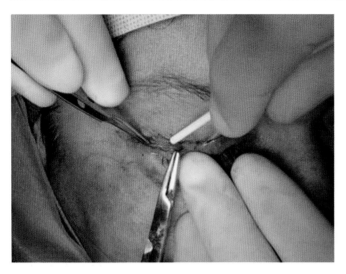

Fig. 15 Running subcuticular closure with mild chromic gut or polypropylene pull-out suture.

Hematoma

Discontinue all antiplatelet and anticoagulation medications appropriately to normalize the patient's coagulation status. Vessels encountered during eyelid surgery can retract into the orbit, and when their integrity is violated, may contribute to postseptal bleeding that may develop into a vision-threatening retrobulbar hematoma. Therefore, control all bleeding points with electrocautery and avoid tugging or excessive tension on the fat pedicle during excision. A retrobulbar hematoma may occlude the central retinal artery and result in vision loss within hours. The patients who present in the postoperative period with swelling, proptosis, pain, and reduced vision should urgently be treated by removal of sutures and/or receive a lateral canthotomy procedure to decompress the hematoma and restore retinal artery blood flow and reduce intraocular pressure. Ophthalmology consultation should be obtained simultaneously with your decompression procedure. Adjunctive therapies include the use of osmotic diuretics, and a head up position to decrease intraocular pressure.

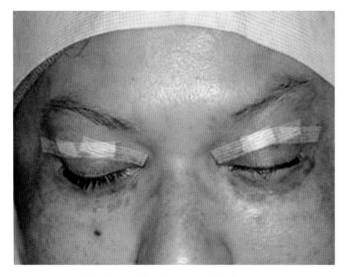

Fig. 16 Adhesive strip skin closure.

Blindness

Blindness is rare and usually related to deep penetration of needles or instruments into the orbit or the development of unrecognized and untreated elevated intraocular pressure secondary to hematoma formation.[12]

Infection

Infection is a rare occurrence following blepharoplasty due to the excellent blood flow and the body's immune surveillance. However, viral herpetic infections are a more likely infectious complication in the susceptible patient experiencing resurfacing.

Dry eye syndrome

The preoperative history and workup will usually elicit dry eye symptoms, and if present, warrant an ophthalmology preoperative referral and consultation. A very conservative periorbital rejuvenation procedure should be considered in these dry eye syndrome patients and procedures should be avoided that may exacerbate the symptoms or adversely affect their ocular health. Some form of methylcellulose eye drops may be necessary postoperatively in this population of patients.

Ptosis

Ptosis usually results from iatrogenic disinsertion of the levator aponeurosis from the tarsal plate and will require a levator suspension procedure to re-establish normal lid position relative to the iris and the superior limbus. A referral to an oculoplastic surgeon for repair is prudent and most appropriate.

Diplopia

Diplopia can result from injury or scarring of the extraocular muscles contributing to the double vision. The most commonly injured extraocular muscles are the superior oblique muscle in the upper eyelid and the inferior oblique muscle in the lower eyelid. Ophthalmology referral will be necessary to address protracted diplopia that does not resolve upon resolution of the postoperative edema.

Scarring

Fortunately, the eyelid skin tends to heal very nicely when surgical principles of tension-free closure and avoidance of incisions outside the envelope of eyelid skin are maintained. If hypertrophic scars develop, massage and intralesional corticosteroid injection usually resolve the patient's concerns.

Asymmetry

It must be remembered that the eyelids are "siblings and not twins." A mild amount of asymmetry is tolerable and expected; however, significant asymmetry, particularly when it comes to crease position, may need to be modified. Usually, the lower lid crease is raised to meet the contralateral higher lid crease. Asymmetric fullness of the eyelids may require re-operation and exploration or the use of neurotoxins, dermal fillers, or resurfacing to correct skin surface asymmetry.

Worsening festoons

Cheek festoons may be exacerbated following certain periorbital invasive procedures that disrupt lymphatic drainage and result in worsening of pre-existing festoons. Worsening of cheek festoons is certainly more likely following lower eyelid procedures, but may on rare occasions be associated with upper eyelid surgery. If the problem occurs and does not seem to be self-limiting once the acute edema resolves, the author has had some success by treating the festoons with a combination of therapies to include laser resurfacing (ablative and nonablative), low-dose corticosteroid (Kenalog) injections, and interestingly, injections of hyaluronidase (Vitrase). There is no science to share regarding the formation of cheek festoons or the rationale for physiologic resolution of the festoons with the therapies mentioned. Anecdotally, these modalities have been effective in the author's hands, and there seems to be a distinct paucity of published evidence-based therapy to achieve resolution of the dreaded cheek festoons.

Periorbital rejuvenation pearls

- Baggy eyelids may herald systemic disease, such as thyroid, renal, or cardiac abnormalities, and will require medical therapy before surgical intervention is contemplated.
- Rule out eyelid ptosis before considering upper eyelid blepharoplasty and refer for ptosis repair before cosmetic surgery of the upper eyelid. Ptosis is a functional disability primarily with a secondary cosmetic concern.
- Address brow position before performing upper eyelid blepharoplasty to avoid making an error in diagnosis that may lead to poor surgical judgment and an unfavorable outcome. Consider surgically addressing the brow and upper eyelid cosmetic concerns simultaneously if you are an experienced facial cosmetic surgeon.
- Be conservative in resective eyelid procedures to avoid undesirable complications. It is always easier to go back and resect more tissue than to attempt replacement of overresected tissues.
- Maintain meticulous hemostasis during eyelid surgery to avoid staining of the tissue planes that may obscure visibility of vital surrounding anatomic structures such as the extraocular muscles that may be subsequently injured resulting in visual disturbances.
- Never overpromise and underdeliver. Show preoperative patients preoperative and postoperative photographs of cases you performed to allow patients to judge your

results to allow you to determine if the patient's expectations are realistic.
- Do not promise significant wrinkle reduction with standard blepharoplasty procedures. These procedures address volume, skin redundancy, and contours without significant changes in skin tone and texture. Resurfacing procedures, neurotoxins, and/or dermal fillers may be required adjunctive procedures to address wrinkles, tone, and texture.
- Many times less is better. Know your own limitations and resist the temptation to go for the "home run" every time. Express your limitations as part of the informed consent process; otherwise, mention of the limitations postoperatively is interpreted as excuses.
- Document your cases with standardized high-resolution clinical photography and always point out defects and asymmetries preoperatively. The patients quickly forget how they looked preoperatively, and photographs provide that documentation accurately and vividly.

References

1. Larrabee WF, Makielski KH. Surgical anatomy of the face. New York: Ravan Press; 1993. p. 129–53.
2. Codner MA, Hanna MK. Applied anatomy of the eyelids and orbit. In: Nahai F, editor. The art of aesthetic surgery-principles and techniques. St Louis (MO): QMP; 2005. p. 626–49.
3. Gunther JP, Antrobus SD. Aesthetic analysis of the eyebrows. Plast Reconstr Surg 1808;99:1997.
4. Nahai F. Clinical decision-making in aesthetic eyelid surgery. In: Nahai F, editor. The art of aesthetic surgery—principles and techniques. St Louis (MO): QMP; 2005. p. 652–78.
5. Flowers RS. Upper blepharoplasty by eyelid invagination. Clin Plast Surg 1993;20:193.
6. Rohrich R. The superficial subciliary cheek lift, a technique for rejuvenating the infraorbital region and the nasojugal groove: a clinical series of 71 patients (discussion). Plast Reconstr Surg 1875;104:199.
7. Pastorek NJ. Blepharoplasty update. Facial Plast Surg Clin North Am 2002;10:23.
8. Saadeh P. Conventional upper and lower blepharoplasty. In: Aston S, Steinbrech DS, Walden JL, editors. Aesthetic plastic surgery. St Louis (MO): Elsevier; 2012. p. 321–8.
9. Codner MA, Hanna MK. Upper and lower blepharoplasty. In: Nahai F, editor. The art of aesthetic surgery—principles and techniques. St Louis (MO): QMP; 2005. p. 680–717.
10. Carruthers J, Carruthers A. Aethetic botulinum A toxin in the mid and lower face and neck. Dermatol Surg 2003;29:468.
11. Lisman RD, Lelli GJ. Treatment of blepharoplasty complications. In: Aston S, Steinbrech DS, Walden JL, editors. Aesthetic plastic surgery. St Louis (MO): Elsevier; 2012. p. 393–408.
12. Stasior OG. Blindness associated with cosmetic blepharoplasty. Clin Plast Surg 1981;8:793.

Lower Transcutaneous Blepharoplasty

Christopher Blake Smith, DMD, MD [a],*, Peter Daniel Waite, MPH, DDS, MD [b]

KEYWORDS

- Periorbital aging • Dermatochalasis • Steatoblepharon • Tear trough deformity • Lower lid malposition

KEY POINTS

- Preoperative planning is crucial to a successful lower eyelid procedure. The surgeon must decide between transconjuctival approach, transcutaneous approach, or a combination of both to address lower lid dermatochalasis and steatoblepharon.
- Lower lid horizontal laxity must be identified before surgery so that it may be properly addressed. This can be accomplished with the eyelid distraction test and the eyelid snap test.
- A deep nasojugal fold or tear trough deformity must be addressed for optimum esthetic outcome. This can be accomplished with the use of fillers, autologous fat grafting, resuspension of orbital fat, or facial implants.

Introduction

Restoration of the aging periorbita to a more refreshed, youthful appearance is arguably one of the most rejuvenating facial cosmetic procedures performed. Blepharoplasty is one of the most frequently performed procedures in the rapidly growing field of cosmetic surgery with more than 200,000 cases documented in 2014, ranking fourth of all procedures. Most patients seeking cosmetic surgery of the lower eyelid are most concerned with dark circles underneath their eyes and "looking tired." A youthful lower eyelid should have a gentle convexity that blends into the upper cheek mound. As the midface ages, periorbital fat can herniate or prolapse through a weakened orbital septum. Known as steatoblepharon or pseudoherniation, this can even be troublesome for young patients (Fig. 1). This, combined with a descent of the malar fat pad, can lead to a double convexity deformity and a deep nasojugal fold.[1] Treatment of the lower eye is aimed at eliminating or tightening redundant skin and muscle, correcting lid laxity, and resecting or redraping retroseptal fat to create a smooth lid-cheek junction (Figs. 2–5). Lower eyelid surgery, however, can be technically challenging, and significant functional defects can result if proper surgical technique and preoperative assessment is not performed.

Preoperative planning

Before any cosmetic surgical procedure, a thorough history and physical examination should be performed. A contraindication to a general surgical procedure is most likely a contraindication to eyelid surgery. Specific to blepharoplasty, ocular history should be elicited from the patient, including history of previous eye surgeries, visual disturbances, use of corrective lenses or contacts, thyroid eye disease, and dry eyes. Lower lid blepharoplasty can be performed in the presence of dry eye syndrome with less risk of potential complications; however, the patient should be informed of the risk before surgery.

To minimize the risk of bleeding, preoperative assessment should include an investigation of medications and herbal supplements that possess anticoagulation properties. Although not an exhaustive list, patients should discontinue aspirin, clopidogrel, nonsteroidals, warfarin, vitamin E, fish oil, and herbal preparations, including St. Johns wort and gingko biloba before surgery. As with any medication, obtain medical consultation as necessary before discontinuation. Alcohol consumption can also increase the risk of bleeding and should be discontinued 2 weeks before surgery.

Horizontal lid laxity should be documented before surgery, because this will guide treatment. Quantitative measures including a snap and distraction test must be documented. A positive lid snap test is defined as greater than 1 second of time elapse for the eyelid returning to its normal position following inferior displacement. The lid distraction test is performed by pulling the lid in an anterior direction away from the globe. Laxity of greater than 6 to 7 mm is considered abnormal, and a lid tightening procedure should be considered (Fig. 6). Lid retraction can be measured quantitatively using margin reflex distance. Margin reflex distance is defined as the distance from the corneal eye reflex to the central portion of the lower lid. Typically this distance is 5 mm with lid retraction increasing this measurement.[2] Simplified, the lower lid should rest at the level of the lower limbus without scleral show. In addition, the surrounding architecture of the periorbita is a predictor of lid position following surgery. Patients with a negative vector as defined by the most anterior portion of the globe lying anterior to the orbital rim are candidates for operative lid support.

Excess or pseudoherniated fat should also be evaluated preoperatively. Gentle ballotement of the globe with the patient in the upright position will determine the location and need for fat removal. Patients should also be evaluated in full

[a] Private Practice, Cosmetic and Facial Surgery of East Alabama, 2971 Corporate Park drive, Opelika, AL 36801, USA
[b] UAB Oral and Maxillofacial Surgery, 1919 7th Avenue South, Birmingham, AL 35233, USA
* Corresponding author.
E-mail address: cblakesmith@gmail.com

Atlas Oral Maxillofacial Surg Clin N Am 24 (2016) 135-145
1061-3315/16/$ - see front matter © 2016 Elsevier Inc. All rights reserved.
http://dx.doi.org/10.1016/j.cxom.2016.05.007

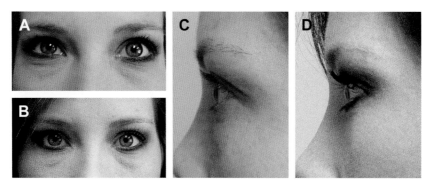

Fig. 1 (*A*) A 28-year-old woman with genetic predisposition to suborbicularis fat herniation. (*B*) 6 weeks following transconjunctival lower blepharoplasty. (*C*) Preoperative left lateral view. (*D*) 6 weeks postoperative left lateral view. Overresection of fat was avoided in this young patient.

smile because hypertrophic orbicularis oculi may be mistaken for excess fat and must be addressed appropriately.

Preparation and patient markings

Standardized and high-quality preoperative and postoperative photographs are an absolute necessity in cosmetic surgery. A standard blepharoplasty series should include full-face frontal, lateral, and three-quarter views as well as close-ups of the same views. In addition, a frontal photograph should be taken with the eyes gazing upward. The authors' preference is to take these photographs at the preoperative appointment with

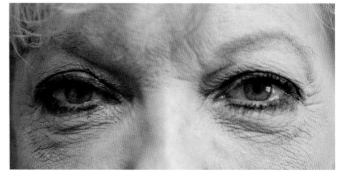

Fig. 3 A 65-year-old woman with significant dermatochalasis and steatoblepharon requiring transcutaneous lower blepharoplasty using skin muscle flap technique.

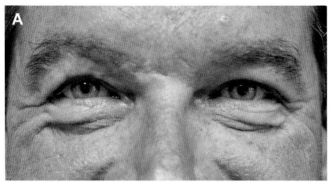

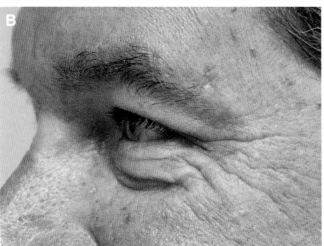

Fig. 2 (*A*, *B*) A 46-year-old man with orbicularis hypertrophy. Orbicularis hypertrophy must be identified preoperatively and addressed with resection orbicularis if indicated.

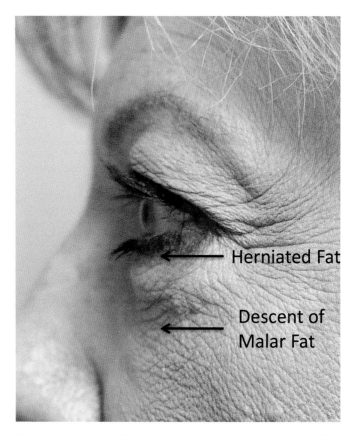

Fig. 4 Herniation of suborbicularis fat as well as descent of the malar fat pad resulting in a double convexity deformity.

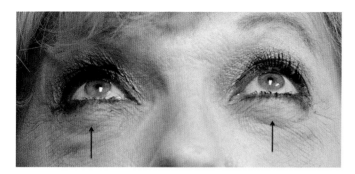

Fig. 5 Asking the patient to look upward will accentuate lower fat pads.

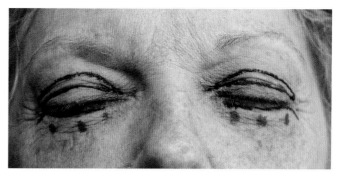

Fig. 7 Preoperative markings for upper blepharoplasty and lower lid subciliary blepharoplasty. The subciliary incision line begins 1 mm lateral to the punctum and extends laterally into the area of an existing rhytid. Suborbicularis fat is marked in green for excision.

makeup on and on day of surgery without makeup. The photographs should also be taken following surgical markings.

Although the patient is in the upright position and in upward gaze, prominent prolapsed orbital fat is marked for removal with an indelible marker. In addition, for the transcutaneous skin muscle flap approach, an incision line is marked 2 to 3 mm inferior to the lash line. This incision should begin 1 mm lateral to the inferior punctum and extend laterally approximately 6 to 8 mm lateral to the lateral canthus. The incision line should be tailored into a lateral rhytid in the area of the crow's feet (Fig. 7). For a skin pinch blepharoplasty, cotton forceps are used to pinch a roll of skin below the lash line, producing slight lash eversion. The redundant tissue is then marked for excision (Fig. 8).

Patient positioning and surgical technique

General anesthesia is preferred for most cosmetic procedures; however, isolated lower lid blepharoplasty can easily be performed with local anesthesia, conscious sedation, or intravenous sedation. Whichever route is used, local anesthesia is a key component. The patient is placed in a supine position before initiation of sedation. One to 2 drops of 0.5% proparacaine or tetracaine ophthalmic are placed into each eye. Corneal eye shields are then placed bilaterally (Fig. 9). Local

anesthesia is injected into the lower eye conjunctiva into medial, central, and lateral fat pads using a 30-gauge needle. A measure of 1% lidocaine (Xylocaine) with 1:100,000 epinephrine can be mixed with a 1:10 dilution of sodium bicarbonate to lessen the initial discomfort of injection through alkalinization of the solution. Local anesthesia should also be injected in a subcutaneous, premuscular plane along the subciliary incision line. If canthopexy/canthoplasty is planned, additional local anesthesia should be injected along the lateral and inferior orbital rim (Fig. 10). The patient is then prepared with betadine or comparable antiseptic solution and draped in sterile fashion. This step allows appropriate time for the hemostatic effect of the epinephrine. If fat grafting is planned, abdominal fat harvest can be performed at this time (Figs. 11 and 12).

Transconjuctival approach

Whether chemical peel, laser skin resurfacing, skin pinch technique, or skin muscle flap approach is taken to address skin laxity of the lower eye, the "prolapsed" or "pseudoherniated" fat is easily addressed through a transconjuctival approach. This approach is used to preserve the middle lamellae as the

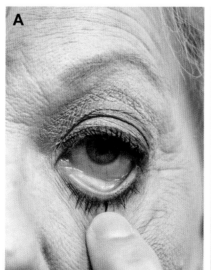
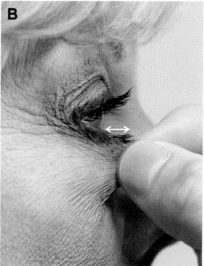

Fig. 6 (*A*) Snap test is performed by inferiorly displacing the lid. The lid should snap back into position in under 1 second. (*B*) The distraction test measures the distance the lid can be distracted from the globe. Less than 6 mm is considered normal.

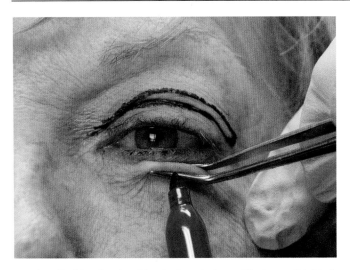

Fig. 8 Marking for the skin pinch technique. The lower lid skin is pinched with cotton forceps until slight lash eversion is seen. This redundant skin is marked for excision.

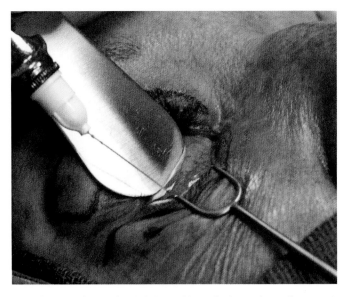

Fig. 10 Local anesthesia injected into the lower lateral, central, and medial fat compartments. Anesthesia is also placed in a subcutaneous plane along the subciliary incision marking.

fat is removed in a retroseptal fashion. The surgeon holds a Jaeger lid plate, and the lower lid is then retracted using a Foman double ball retractor held by the assistant. Alternatively, a Desmarres lid retractor may be used for lower lid eversion. The lid plate is used to exert gentle pressure on the globe, making the prolapsed fat more evident. The incision is made approximately 8 mm posterior to the eyelid margin, avoiding the tarsal plate. This incision can be accomplished with needle point electrocautery on cut setting, radiofrequency technology, or CO_2 laser. The incision is made from the puctum medially to the lateral canthus laterally. A continuous motion is used to incise through the conjunctiva and capsulopalpebral fascia (Fig. 13). Following the incision, the assistant then controls the lid plate as well as the lid retractor, affording the surgeon both hands to gently tease out the fat with fine Adson forceps and incise along the surrounding capsule with electrocautery. The fat is excised using electrocautery on coagulation setting, radiofrequency, or CO_2 laser. The central fat pad often herniates through the incision and is easily removed. A fine hemostat may be required to gently allow the medial and lateral fat pads to become evident. Care must be taken to protect the inferior oblique muscle because it lies between the medial and central fat pads. The surgeon should periodically remove all instrumentation, and with gentle ballottement of the globe, evaluate appropriate and symmetric fat removal. Conservative fat excision is key to an

esthetic result as overresection can result in a hollowed out appearance. Only fat that freely herniates into the incision or teases out with gentle traction is indicated for removal. Once adequate fat removal is accomplished, the surgeon must address the skin laxity in the lower eyelid. Further discussion will be limited to the transcutaneous approaches because other techniques are discussed in another article (see Sean Pack, Faisal A. Quereshy, Mehmet Ali Altay, et al, "Transconjunctival Lower Blepharoplasty," in this issue).

Skin pinch technique

Most patients undergoing lower eyelid blepharoplasty are excellent candidates for less invasive skin tightening techniques such as laser skin resurfacing or chemical peel to address skin laxity and fine rhytids. There is a subset of patients that have excessive dermatochalasis that will not be adequately treated with laser or peels alone. Another subset of patients are not candidates for laser skin resurfacing due to pigmented skin or do not desire the prolonged erythema of laser treatment. These patients are indicated for transcutaneous techniques and will appreciate maximum esthetic outcome.

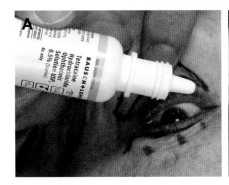
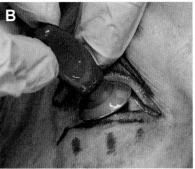

Fig. 9 (A) 0.5% Tetracaine placed into eye. (B) Stainless steel corneal protectors inserted using suction cup.

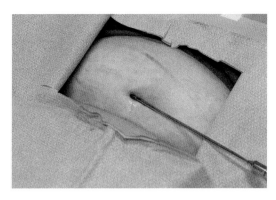

Fig. 11 Abdominal fat harvested using standard liposuction cannula through umbilical punctures. Fat is harvested into 20-mL syringe. Before harvest, approximately 500-mL of tumescent fluid was injected.

Skin pinch technique is a simple procedure ideally performed in conjunction with transconjunctival blepharoplasty. This technique is designed to preserve the orbital septum as the fat is harvested from a retroseptal approach. During preoperative patient marking, lower eyelid skin is pinched with cotton forceps to produce slight lash eversion. Once adequate skin excision is determined, it is marked with an indelible marker.

Following transconjuctival blepharoplasty, no additional local anesthesia is typically required to perform the skin pinch technique, because this tends to distort the tissue. A curved hemostat can be used to crimp the tissue below the lash line in the preoperative marking and will result in a raised line of excess skin with a crushed base. The elevated skin is then excised with sharp curved iris or Westcott scissors. The crushing effect of the hemostat produces a hemostatic effect, and minimal bleeding is encountered. Alternatively, a Brown-Adson forceps can be used to pinch the skin in the lateral, central, and medial regions to mark the excess. Approximately 3 to 5 mm of skin is generally excised. Excess orbicularis muscle can be trimmed if indicated; however, the surgeon should consider a skin muscle flap approach to address orbicularis hypertrophy. Closure is performed with 6-0 fast absorbing gut sutures in a running fashion (Fig. 14).

Skin-muscle flap approach

The skin-muscle flap approach is a safe procedure traditionally performed to address orbicularis oculi hypertrophy and excess lower eyelid skin. Pseudoherniated orbital fat can also be addressed through this approach; however, orbital septum must be violated. This approach does have the potential for ectropion, lid retraction, and scleral show if excess skin is resected or if pretarsal orbicularis is not preserved. In the past, this was considered the universal approach and often resulted in an overoperated appearance. The novice surgeon must be cognizant of these potential complications and understand the management if such problem should arise. Selecting the correct procedure for the right patient is of paramount importance.

Incision and flap elevation

A subciliary incision is marked 2 to 3 mm below the lash line before initiation of sedation or injection of local anesthesia. This incision line begins 1 mm lateral to the inferior punctum and extends 6 to 8 mm lateral to the lateral canthus. The incision line is tailored into one of the existing crow's feet. If upper blepharoplasty is also planned, 5 to 10 mm of intact skin should exist between the 2 markings (Fig. 15). This intact skin will minimize risk of prolonged lymphedema.

Following initiation of sedation or general anesthesia, local anesthesia is injected in a subcutaneous plane along the subciliary incision line. A No. 15 surgical blade is then used to make an incision in the previous surgical marking. A Frost stitch using a 5-0 Nylon suture may then be placed in the tarsal plate just lateral to the lateral limbus for retraction (Fig. 16). Depending on the preoperative assessment, a skin-only flap to the last wrinkle may be all that is required for correction of dermatochalasis. If orbicularis redundancy or flaccidity exists, the surgeon must proceed with a skin-muscle flap.[3] A skin-only flap is raised for approximately 6 to 8 mm preserving the pretarsal orbicularis. Preserving this cuff of orbicularis will minimize risk of ectropion and lower lid laxity following surgery (Fig. 17). An incision is then made in the orbicularis oculi muscle and dissection continues inferiorly in a relatively avascular plane just superior to the orbital septum down to the level of the orbital rim.

Orbital fat management

At this point, buttonhole incisions may be made in the orbital septum, and medial, central, and lateral fat pads may be excised. To minimize risk of bleeding, this can be performed with electrocautery. Many advocate injection of local anesthesia into individual fat pads; however, some feel this is unnecessary and may cause rebound bleeding. Alternatively, the surgeon may choose to redrape the fat to correct a tear trough

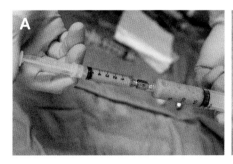
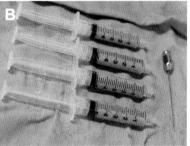

Fig. 12 (*A*) Harvested fat is set aside and allowed to separate. The infranatant tumescent fluid is discarded, and the supernatant fat is transferred into 5-mL syringes using a female-to-female transfer. (*B*) Fat ready for injection using microcannula.

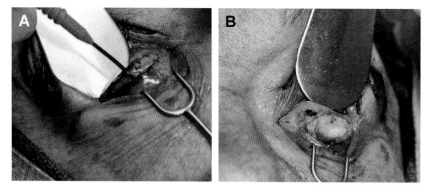

Fig. 13 (*A*) Lower transconjunctival incision using electrocautery on cut setting. This is done with a continuous sweeping motion through the conjunctiva and capsulopalpebral fascia. (*B*) The central fat herniating through the incision.

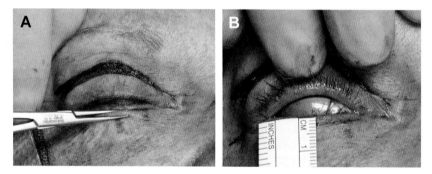

Fig. 14 (*A*) A fine hemostat is used to crush tissue for the skin pinch technique. This will aid in hemostasis, and the raised redundant skin is excised and closed with 6-0 gut suture. (*B*) For skin muscle flap technique, the incision is placed 3 to 4 mm below the lash line.

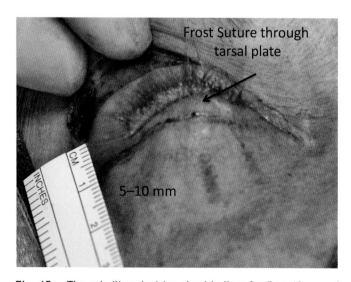

Fig. 15 The subciliary incision should allow for 5 to 10 mm of intact skin between the upper blepharoplasty incision. A Frost stitch is placed through the tarsal plate to aid in retraction and protection of the globe.

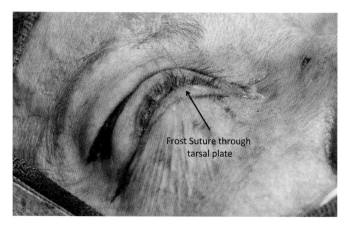

Fig. 16 Frost suture placed in lower tarsus for retraction and protection of the globe.

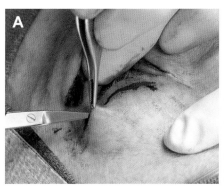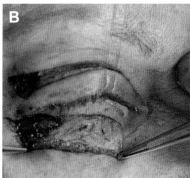

Fig. 17 (*A*) Development of the skin-only flap protecting the 4 to 5 mm of pretarsal orbicularis for lower lid support. (*B*) Skin flap elevated before division of the orbicularis muscle. Dissection will then proceed to the orbital rim in a preseptal plane.

deformity. For this approach, dissection proceeds inferiorly below the orbital rim in a preperiosteal plane for approximately 1.5 to 2 cm to create a pocket in the region of the tear trough. The medial and central fat pads are secured to the periosteum with a 6-0 Vicryl suture. The lateral fat pad is almost always excised and not redraped.

Orbicularis oculi muscle

Once the skin muscle flap has been developed, an orbicularis sling provides additional support to the lid and provides a subtle malar lift. Similar to the procedure described by Hamra,[4] a laterally based pendant of orbicularis is secured to the lateral orbital rim through the upper blepharoplasty incision and is accomplished using a 4-0 Prolene suture attached to the lateral orbital rim. The suture is then tunneled to the orbicularis oculi muscle in the lateral aspect of the skin muscle flap. This technique adds significant support to the flap and allows passive draping of the excess skin (Fig. 18).

Lower lid support

Multiple algorithms for treatment of horizontal lid laxity have been described. One should distinguish between mild-to-moderate lid laxity and severe laxity based on snap and distraction tests. If lid laxity was noted preoperatively from a positive snap test or lid distraction of 6 mm, it can be

addressed at this time with a lateral canthopexy. Similar to Fagien's approach,[5] a 4-0 Polyglactin (Vicryl) suture can be passed from the upper blepharoplasty incision through the lateral retinaculum of the lower lid in a horizontal mattress fashion. The suture is returned to the upper blepharoplasty incision and secured to the internal lateral orbital rim (Fig. 19). The vector of pull should result in narrowing of the lateral canthal angle and movement in a superior lateral direction as well as adapting the lid to the globe. According to McCord and colleagues,[6] severe lid laxity is greater than 6 mm of anterior lid distraction. The authors prefer to treat this with a lid-shortening canthoplasty. A wedge excision of the lateral lower eyelid is performed with iris scissors and secured in a similar fashion to the internal lateral orbital rim.

Skin excision

The excess skin is draped passively over the incision line and excised with curved iris or Westcott scissors. The vector of pull is in a superior medial direction (Fig. 20). The scissors may be turned with the beaks down for the final extent of the excision, resulting in a nicely tailored excision and facilitates closure (Fig. 21). The skin is then closed with a 6-0 fast absorbing gut suture in a running fashion. At this time, fat can be grafted in the tear troughs, malar, and submalar regions as desired (Fig. 22). Following the completion of the procedure, corneal eye shields are removed, and the eyes are rinsed with a balanced salt solution (Figs. 23–26).

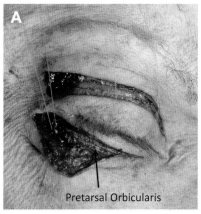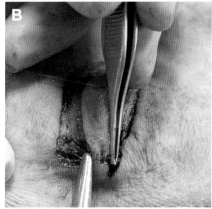

Fig. 18 (*A*) Orbicularis sling procedure providing lid support. Prolene suture is used to suspend preseptal orbicularis to the lateral orbital rim. (*B*) The Prolene is tunneled to the lateral orbital rim.

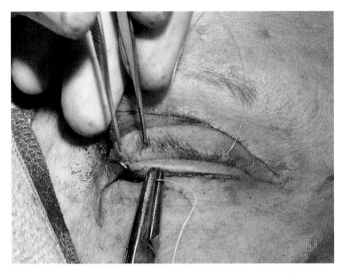

Fig. 19 Canthopexy to tighten the laxity in the lower lid. Lateral retinaculum is secured to the internal lateral orbital rim using Vicryl suture.

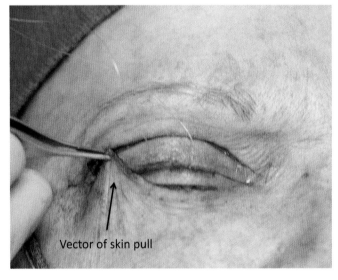

Fig. 20 The skin is allowed to drape passively following the orbicularis sling. When trimming excess skin, the pull with the Adson forceps is in a superior medial direction.

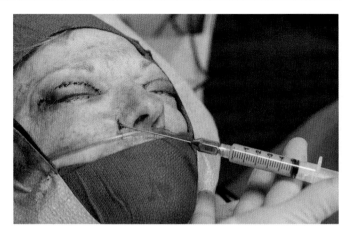

Fig. 22 Harvested abdominal fat is grafted into the tear troughs, submalar region, and malar region in a subperiosteal plane.

Complications

As with any surgery, complications are not always preventable, and the surgeon must be prepared to manage them as they arise. Serious complications can largely be avoided through proper patient selection, meticulous surgical technique, and proper postoperative care. Patients must also be educated before surgery regarding a normal postoperative course of potential temporary blurry vision, edema, ecchymosis, eyelid numbness, and dry eyes. These postoperative problems are not considered complications, and patient reassurance is usually the only treatment required.

Bleeding

Retrobulbar hemorrhage with associated vision loss is the most feared and serious complication following cosmetic eyelid surgery. Fortunately, this is an extremely rare complication with the most recent literature estimating the incidence of orbital hemorrhage at 1:2000 (0.05%) and hemorrhage with permanent vision loss at 1:10,000 (0.01%).[7] However, the surgeon must quickly recognize this potential complication and understand its management. The patient will typically present within the first 24 hours following surgery with extreme pain, signs of vision loss, tense protruding orbit, decreased ocular motility, and a relative afferent pupillary defect. If a tonometer pen is available, ocular pressure should be measured.

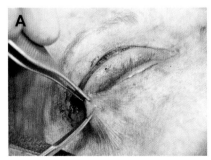
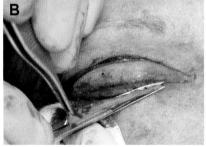

Fig. 21 (*A*) The excess lower lid skin is trimmed. (*B*) Flipping the beaks for the final excision results in a crisp excision line that facilitates cosmetic closure.

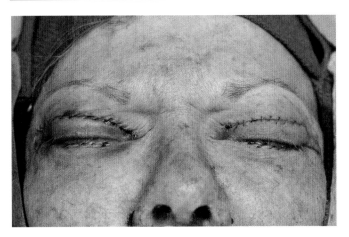

Fig. 23 Immediately following upper and lower skin muscle flap blepharoplasty with fat grafting.

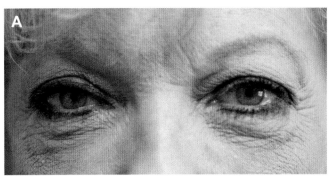

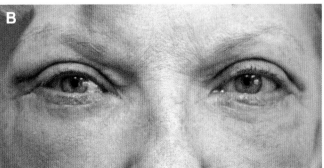

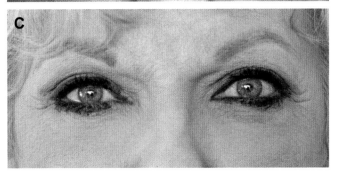

Intraocular pressure greater than 40 mm Hg requires emergent treatment with lateral canthotomy and inferior cantholysis to decompress the orbital contents. Prompt ophthalmologic consultation is also imperative. A tonometer pen is also useful at differentiating an ocular emergency from postoperative bleeding and swelling resulting in a tense protruding orbit. In this case, the surgeon may decide to monitor and allow swelling to resolve with time.[8]

Intraoperative control of bleeding is best handled with meticulous surgical technique. Monopolar or bipolar cautery is essential to the blepharoplasty surgeon to control brisk bleeding. Many surgeons recommend clamping fat pads and injection of local anesthetic before excision. It is the authors' preference to identify vessels and cauterize directly during the excision rather than relying on the hemostatic effect of epinephrine and force of the hemostat.

Lower eyelid malposition

Lower eyelid malposition following blepharoplasty is a potentially serious complication and can range from mild scleral show and canthal rounding to frank ectropion with lower lid eversion. Lower lid descent and retraction is multifactorial, including untreated preoperative lateral canthal tendon laxity, anterior lamellae insufficiency from excess skin excision, middle lamellae scarring between the orbital septum and capsulopalpebral fascia, and malar descent. Common problems

Fig. 25 (*A*) Preoperative, (*B*) 1 week following upper and lower transcutaneous blepharoplasty with fat grafting, (*C*) 6 weeks postoperative.

arise from excessive muscle suturing and aggressive repositioning lid anatomy. Small changes in eyelid anatomy are often profound. Mild scleral show and lid retraction can be conservatively managed with ocular lubrication and massage. An alternative is release of sutures in the early postoperative period, leaving an open wound. This open wound may result in an unaesthetic wound, and delayed skin grafting may be

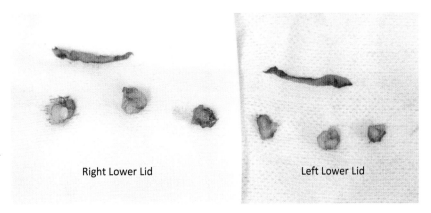

Right Lower Lid   Left Lower Lid

Fig. 24 It is important to document tissue removed for symmetry and record keeping.

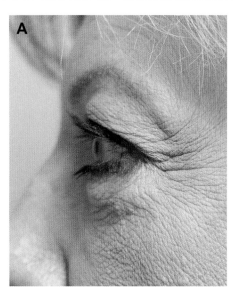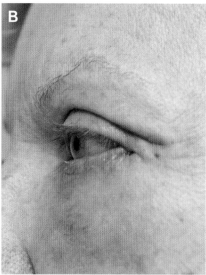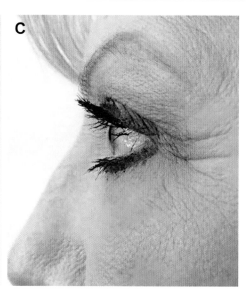

Fig. 26   (A) Preoperative, (B) 1 week following upper and lower transcutaneous blepharoplasty with fat grafting, (C) 6 weeks postoperative.

necessary. In the case of extreme malposition or failure of conservative measures, surgical intervention is necessary including skin grafts for anterior lamellae lengthening and mucosal grafts for posterior lamellae lengthening. Canthopexy or tarsal strip procedures may also be necessary to correct lid malposition.

Chemosis

Although a relatively minor complication, chemosis can be disconcerting to patients. Edema of the conjunctiva can be impressive, and steroids are typically indicated for these cases. Typically treatment with methylprednisolone taper as well as Tobramycin/Dexamethasone ophthalmic is adequate. Chemosis is generally self-limiting and refractory cases may warrant referral to ophthalmologist.

Dry eyes

Although not as common a complication with lower lid blepharoplasty, dry, irritated eyes can be annoying to patients. Prevention is aimed at hydration, lubrication, and minimizing edema. Dry eyes can typically be managed with ophthalmic lubricants and artificial tears until resolution.

Postoperative care

Postoperative care is relatively simple following lower transcutaneous blepharoplasty. Patients are instructed to rest with head elevated and avoid lifting anything greater than 10 pounds for a week. These instructions are aimed at minimizing elevations in blood pressure. Patients currently treated for hypertension are instructed to continue antihypertensives as prescribed. For the first 24 to 48 hours, patients are instructed to keep cold packs on the area as much as possible. Keeping cold packs on the area can be accomplished with crushed ice, iced saline gauze, Swiss eye therapy, frozen peas, or chilled washcloths. Whatever modality is chosen, as long as the

patient is adherent to the protocol, will work so that swelling can be reduced.[9]

Minimal antibiotic ointment is indicated for the subciliary or skin pinch incision for a week as well as a systemic antibiotic to cover skin flora for 24 hours. Keflex or similar cephalosporin as well as Bacitracin or Polysporin is generally acceptable. Tobramycin/Dexamethasone ophthalmic and methylprednisolone taper can be prescribed as needed if severe chemosis or allergic eyes occur. Some surgeons advocate the routine use of steroid tapers or ophthalmic ointments; however, this is not typically necessary. Pain is fairly minimal following blepharoplasty and can usually be managed with nonsteroidal medications. Narcotics are typically written for breakthrough pain. Benzodiazepines for patient comfort following cosmetic surgery are often beneficial.

Follow-up care

Patients are seen on postoperative day 1 to evaluate for early potential problems such as hematoma, corneal abrasion, or abnormal swelling. Patients are again seen at 1 week, when any residual sutures are removed and reassurance is given regarding progress. Patients are then allowed to heal for 6 weeks, and postoperative photographs are taken at this appointment. In general, blepharoplasty patients are pleased with their results. It is at this appointment that preoperative photographs can be evaluated for patients that fail to see the improvement. The final follow-up is done at 3 months, and any potential complications such as lid malposition or poor scarring can be addressed.

Summary

Treatment of the aging periorbita can be extremely rewarding for surgeon and patient. Lower transcutaneous blepharoplasty can be a daunting procedure to the novice surgeon due to the potential serious complications. Proper patient selection, a conservative approach, as well as adhering to strict surgical principles allows the novice surgeon to gain experience and advance their skills.

References

1. Crumley RL, Torkian BA, Karam AM. Lower eyelid blepharoplasty. Facial plastic and reconstructive surgery. 3rd edition. New York: Thieme; 2009. p. 271–85.
2. Fattahi T. Blepharoplasty. Fonseca oral and maxillofacial surgery. 2nd edition, vol. 3. St Louis (MO): Saunders/Elsevier; 2009. p. 579–94.
3. de Castro CC. A critical analysis of the current surgical concepts for lower blepharoplasty. Plast Reconstr Surg 2004;114(3):785–93 [discussion: 794–6].
4. Hamra ST. The role of orbital fat preservation in facial aesthetic surgery. A new concept. Clin Plast Surg 1996;23(1):17–28.
5. Fagien S. Algorithm for canthoplasty: the lateral retinacular suspension: a simplified suture canthopexy. Plast Reconstr Surg 1999; 103(7):2042–53 [discussion: 2054–8].
6. McCord CD, Boswell CB, Hester TR. Lateral canthal anchoring. Plast Reconstr Surg 2003;112(1):222–37 [discussion: 238–9].
7. Hass AN, Penne RB, Stefanyszyn MA, et al. Incidence of post-blepharoplasty orbital hemorrhage and associated visual loss. Ophthal Plast Reconstr Surg 2004;20:426–32.
8. Niamtu J III. Cosmetic blepharoplasty. Facial cosmetic surgery. St Louis (MO): Elsevier; 2011. p. 129–74.
9. Walrath JD, Hayek BR, Wojno T. Blepharoplasty. Current therapy in oral and maxillofacial surgery. St Louis (MO): Saunders/Elsevier; 2012. p. 986–95.

Transconjunctival Lower Blepharoplasty

Sean Pack, DDS, MD [a], Faisal A. Quereshy, MD, DDS [a],*,
Mehmet Ali Altay, DDS, PhD [b], Dale A. Baur, DDS [a]

KEYWORDS

- Lid—cheek junction • Tear trough • Transconjunctival approach • Fat repositioning

KEY POINTS

- With lower blepharoplasties, there is no secret to achieving successful results; as is the case with any surgical procedure, proper patient evaluation and development of a comprehensive, anatomic-based treatment plan are prerequisites for success.
- For situations in which a patient has little lid laxity and pseudoherniated periorbital fat, transconjunctival lower blepharoplasty is the treatment of choice.
- Transconjunctival lower blepharoplasty enables the surgeon to reposition fat, effectively blending the lid—cheek junction and filling the tear trough deformity.
- In order to better enable clinicians to achieve optimal outcomes, the authors advocate an anatomic-based approach for patient evaluation and treatment planning.

Introduction

"The eyes are the windows to the soul." although somewhat cliché, this proverb is meaningful for the cosmetic surgeon. As a part of the human experience, it is settled fact that the eyes play an important role in both verbal and nonverbal communication; they convey the full range of human emotions. In light of this, many patients seek to alter the appearance of their eyes or, more specifically, their lower eyelids. There are a number of reasons why patients often seek lower eyelid rejuvenation. In the authors' experience, some of the most common reasons have been for correction of a tired, aged, or sad appearance.

Despite being an often-requested procedure, many surgeons have completely abandoned performing lower blepharoplasty due to the frequency of complications and their potentially devastating nature. It is the authors' belief that most of these complications are avoidable. With a proper knowledge of lower eyelid anatomy and the pathophysiology of aging, and the development of a logical guide for treatment planning, it is possible to predictably perform transconjunctival lower blepharoplasty. As such, the purpose of this article is to equip the clinician with knowledge of the indications and technical details of the transconjunctival lower blepharoplasty. In doing so, the authors hope to give confidence to the cosmetic surgeon and improve his or her chances of success.

Anatomy

To properly treat patients with aged lower eyelids, one must have a well-founded understanding of lower eyelid anatomy.

This is prerequisite for development of an anatomic-based treatment plan. To proceed without this knowledge will invariably lead to unpredictable outcomes.

Before describing the organization of the periorbital soft tissues, it is necessary to understand the dimensions of the bony orbit and its contents. As a general rule, the bony orbit is conical in shape, with a depth of 38 to 44 mm, a height of 33 to 37 mm, and a width of 38 to 41 mm.[1] On average, the internal volume of the orbit is approximately 30 cc and is filled with the following structures: the globe (10 cc), extraocular muscles (10 cc), and orbital fat and lacrimal gland (10 cc).[1,2]

Of particular interest in lower blepharoplasty is the organization of periorbital fat. Postseptal orbital fat is organized into 5 discrete pads, 2 upper and 3 lower pads. With regard to the 3 lower fat pads, there is a lateral, middle, and medial fat pad. Of note, the middle and medial fat pads are connected by a narrow isthmus of fat and are separated by the inferior oblique muscle.[3]

In addition to being organized into fat pads, orbital fat is also unevenly distributed within the orbit, with the majority being located posteriorly, in supraperiosteal pockets between intramuscular septae. In fact, approximately 60% to 70% of the fat volume is located deep within the bony orbit, posterior to the globe. As a result, posterior orbital fat has relatively little effect on vertical globe support. This function primarily belongs to the aforementioned orbital fat pads. This concept is important, as removal of only a small amount of orbital fat from the anterior areas, those immediately deep to the orbital septum, can have a profound effect on globe position. In 1986, Manson demonstrated that removal of 0.5 cc (a pea-sized volume) of orbital fat caused the globe to move 1 mm inferiorly and 2 mm posteriorly.[1,4,5] This highlights the authors' position that orbital fat should either be repositioned or, at most, removed judiciously.

Now that the contents of the bony orbit have been discussed, one is in a better position to examine the organization

[a] Department of Oral and Maxillofacial Surgery, Case Western Reserve University, 2124 Cornell Road, Room DOA 53A, Cleveland, OH 44106, USA
[b] Department of Oral and Maxillofacial Surgery, Akdeniz University, Antalya, Turkey
* Corresponding author.
E-mail address: faq@case.edu

Atlas Oral Maxillofacial Surg Clin N Am 24 (2016) 147-151
1061-3315/16/$ - see front matter © 2016 Elsevier Inc. All rights reserved.
http://dx.doi.org/10.1016/j.cxom.2016.05.011

of the periorbital soft tissues. The periorbital soft tissues of the eyelid are described in layered/lamellar terms, with an anterior and a posterior lamella separated by the orbital septum (Fig. 1). From superficial to deep, the anterior lamella is composed of skin, subcutaneous adipose tissue (ie, malar fat), and orbicularis muscle. This muscle is divided into 3 discrete components: pretarsal orbicularis (overlying the inferior tarsal plate), preseptal (overlying orbital septum), and preorbital (overlying the facial bones) (Fig. 2).[6] The fibrous attachment of the orbicularis is at the lateral orbital rim, at a discrete fibrous structure termed the lateral thickening. Extending medially from the lateral thickening, along the inferior rim, is another ligament of import, the orbicular retaining ligament (ORL). This ligament attaches the orbicularis muscle to the zygomatic bone. Knowledge of the function and location of this structure is a prerequisite to understanding the pathophysiology of lower lid aging, which will be discussed later. Next, immediately deep to the orbicularis muscle is the orbital septum, which separates the anterior and posterior lamella. With regard to the posterior lamella, it is composed of the inferior tarsus and palpebral conjunctiva.[6]

With an understanding of layered organization of the periorbital soft tissues, one can discuss a key component of the globe's support apparatus, the lateral canthal tendon (LCT). With regard to the LCT, it has 2 main support functions. First, it provides lateral anchorage for the eyelids, and, second it provides vertical support for the globe and lower lid. The bony attachment of the LCT is at Whitnall tubercle, located approximately 4 mm posterior to the lateral orbital rim, on the lateral orbital wall.[7,8] It is from this site that the LCT extends inferomedially, attaching to the lateral aspects of the upper and lower tarsal plates. In addition, the LCT is situated 2 to 3 mm superior to the medial canthal tendon. This helps form a 2 to 3° tilted intercanthal axis, a desirable characteristic.[9]

Pathophysiology of aging

Lower eyelid aging, like all physiologic processes, is the result of cause-and-effect relationships. The cumulative effect of these relationships results in common and well-documented physical findings. In this section, the precise cause of many of

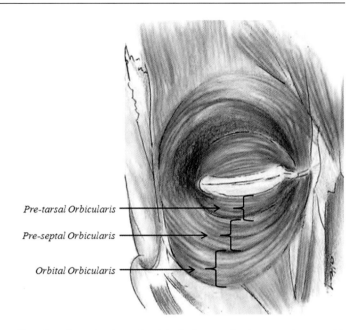

Fig. 2 Organization of orbicularis muscle in accordance with underlying anatomical structures.

physical examination findings common to aged lower eyelids will be discussed. This will better enable the surgeon to address the source of a patient's chief complaint, improving the likelihood of a successful outcome.[1,9]

The anatomic discussion of lower-lid changes will begin with the external appearance of the aged lower eyelid. One of the most common findings is often described as puffy eyelids. This finding represents the merger of the lid–cheek junction with the tear trough (Fig. 3). Merger of these discrete entities forms a continuous furrow that delineates displaced/pseudoherniated postseptal fat from inferiorly displaced, sagging, suborbicularis oculi fat (SOOF) pad. The end result of these anatomic changes is development lower lid bags, which represent herniated or, more commonly, pseudoherniated postseptal fat.[1,10]

With regard to the surface appearance of the lateral lower eyelid, there are other noteworthy changes. First among them is the presence of fine rhytids and crow's feet extending from the lateral canthus. These findings are often the result of ultraviolet (UV) damage in conjunction with an age-related decrease in collagen remodeling. In addition to development of fine rhytids and crow's feet, the lateral canthal angle also becomes more rounded with age. This is the result of increased laxity of the LCT. The end result of this age-related process is loss of the aesthetic, almond-shaped palpebral aperture, ectropion, increased scleral show, and generalized accentuation of lower lid rhytids.[1,11]

Each of the aforementioned physical findings has interconnected etiologies. As such, the authors next describe the lower lid aging process as a chain reaction, the first step of which is the development of progressive laxity of the globe support apparatus, which is primarily comprised of Lockwood suspensory ligament (LL) and the LCT (Fig. 4). As a consequence, the globe descends and translates posteriorly, displacing postseptal fat anteriorly, leading it to bulge/pseudoherniate through the orbital septum (Fig. 5). This process accounts for both lower lid bags and sunken eyes. In addition, increased laxity of the LCT and LL not only displaces

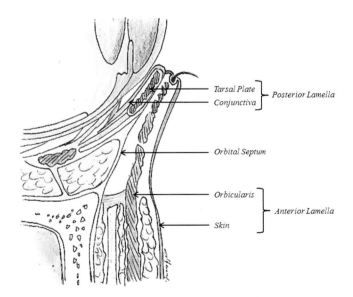

Fig. 1 Lamellar organization of periorbital soft tissues.

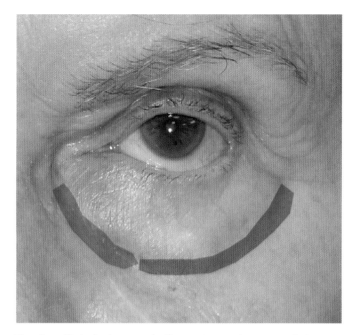

Fig. 3 Clinical photograph illustrating coalescence of the tear trough deformity and the lid—cheek junction in the aged lower eyelid. The blue highlighted area represents the tear trough deformity, which is bordered by 3 muscles: levator palpebrae superioris, levator palpebrae superioris alequae nasae, and the orbicularis muscles. The gray highlighted area represents the lid—cheek junction, formed by the ORL's containment of pseudoherniated postseptal fat. Note the presence of the lower lid bag, ectropion, increased scleral show, and rounded lateral aspect of the orbital aperture.

the globe and postseptal fat, but also leads to shortening of the palpebral aperture, ectropion, and accentuated rhytids.[9]

As stated earlier, the senile development of LCT and LL laxity starts a chain of events that leads to many unaesthetic periorbital soft tissue changes. One of the more distressing

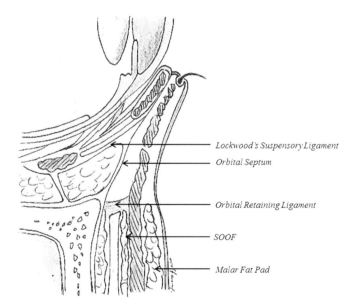

Fig. 4 Sagittal representation of the lower lid and periorbital soft tissues.

Lockwood's Suspensory Ligament

Orbital Septum

Orbital Retaining Ligament

SOOF

Malar Fat Pad

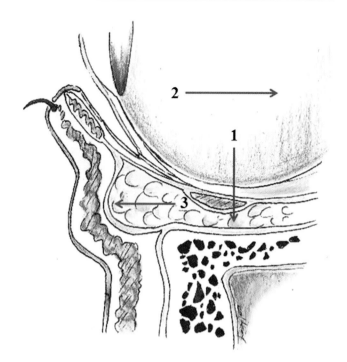

Fig. 5 Stepwise process of lower lid fat pseudoherniation. Step 1: development of increased laxity of the LCT and LL with subsequent loss of vertical globe support and inferior displacement of the globe. Steps 2 and 3: posterior globe translation, which displaces postseptal fat forward.

changes is development of the aforementioned lower lid bag. This defect results in dark circles as a consequence of shadowing. The bulk of the infraorbital bulge is caused by displaced postseptal fat that bulges anteriorly, with the inferior margin of the bulge being contained by the ORL. This association forms the all-important lid—cheek junction.[1,11,12]

Confluent with the lid—cheek junction is another common age-related lower lid abnormality, the tear trough deformity (see Fig. 3). Unlike the lid—cheek junction, however, the tear trough deformity does not owe its genesis to increased LCT laxity. On the contrary, it results from descent of the malar fat pad and exposure of a triangular intermuscular depression. The following muscles border this depression: levator palpebrae superioris, levator palpebrae superioris alequae nasae, and the orbicualis.[5,7,8]

Finally, as people age, the aforementioned orbital fat pads do not increase in volume. In fact, there is a tendency for lipoatrophy.[1] In other words, the characteristic infraorbital fat bags that are common with aging are not caused by an increase in adipose volume.[1] They are actually caused by changes in globe position and periorbital fat distribution. This is pertinent when developing a treatment plan for the patient with lower eyelid fat pseudoherniation. This condition is properly treated with fat repositioning.[12] In the authors' experience, a transconjunctival approach with globe resuspension and lateral canthopexy is effective.

Indications

Like any cosmetic procedure, the use of the transcutaneous blepharoplasty has specific indications. One particular indication is for the patient with pseudoherniated fat, minimal-to-moderate moderate skin laxity, and minimal orbicularis

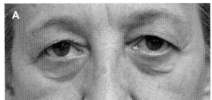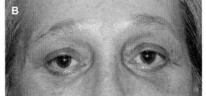

Fig. 6   Preoperative (*A*) and 4-week postoperative (*B*) photos of a 59-year-old woman after transconjunctival lower blepharoplasty with a skin pinch excision and lateral canthopexy.

redundancy. However, these indications are not absolute. In fact, the transcutaneous approach may be utilized in conjunction with other adjunctive procedures (ie, skin pinch and lateral canthopexy), making it a versatile technique (Fig. 6).

Advantages and disadvantages

Now that the surgical anatomy of the orbit, the pathophysiology of aging, and the indications of use have been described, one is better prepared to understand the advantages and disadvantages of the transconjunctival lower blepharoplasty. First, the advantages, which are numerous, will be discussed. Chief among them is a decrease in incidence of 1 of the major complications of transcutaneous lower blepharoplasties, ectropion. Limiting the incision to the conjunctiva and avoiding dissection of the delicate anterior lamella vastly reduce the risk of scar contracture of the lower lid.[11] In addition, the transconjunctival approach eliminates visible scarring.

In most cases, the advantages of the transconjunctival approach outweigh the disadvantages; however, this is not always the case. For instance, patients with excessive lid laxity often warrant a transcutaneous approach with skin and muscle resection. Another shortcoming of the transconjunctival approach is the higher level of technical skill required.

Technique

Because of its versatility, transconjunctival fat repositioning has become one of the most commonly used techniques in lower blepharoplasty. This approach is indicated for patients with lower lid bags and minimal-to-moderate skin laxity. Another common finding is a prominent lid–cheek junction/ lower lid bag, which can be addressed with this procedure alone, or in combination with a midface lift.

After intubation, the lower lid is retracted anteriorly using a 5-0 prolene tarsal stitch. At this point, with the lower lid retracted anteriorly, the authors administer approximately 3 cc of 1% lidocaine 1:100 K epinephrine in the subconjunctival plane and in the subcutaneous plane near the LCT. Next, they complete a standard lateral canthotomy.

At this point, the conjunctiva is incised 1 to 2 mm inferior to the tarsal plate using bovie electrocautery (Fig. 7). This incision extends medially along the length of the lower lid, stopping 5 mm lateral to the medial punctum. The incision is carried to a depth superficial to the orbital septum. One should see the orbicularis muscle at the depth of the incision. Once the orbicularis is exposed within the length of the incision, this plane is developed inferiorly using curved Metzenbaum scissors to the inferior orbital rim. At the level of the orbital rim, and consequently the arcus marginalis, the arcus is incised with a

bovie to the level of the orbital rim (Fig. 8). This dissection is continued in a subperiosteal plane 5 mm inferior to the arcus marginalis (see Fig. 8). This effectively lyses the ligamentous attachment of the orbicularis oculi muscle to the midfacial skeleton. At the same level, this dissection is carried medially into the tear trough. These steps are critical, as they will form the pocket into which the periorbital fat will be repositioned.

At this point, one is prepared to reposition the pseudo-herniated orbital fat over the inferior orbital rim, into the previously dissected subperiosteal pocket. To begin this process, the orbital fat is gently teased out, over the rim, using a curved hemostat (see Fig. 8). Next, using 5-0 vicryl suture on a tapered P-3 needle, the fat is tacked to periosteum at the depth of the subperiosteal dissection, inferior to the attachment of the arcus, and into the tear–trough deformity. This technique effectively blends the lid–cheek junction. Finally, closure is completed with 4 interrupted 6-0 fast absorbable gut sutures in the palpebral conjunctiva.[13,14]

In the authors' practice, prophylactic lateral canthopexy is nearly always implemented in conjunction with lower blepharoplasty. By superiorly positioning the LCT, this simple and quick adjunct improves globe support and tightens lower lid skin.[14] To begin this portion of the procedure, toothed tissue forceps are used to grasp the common limb of the LCT, which was lysed in the initial steps of this procedure. A 5-0 nylon

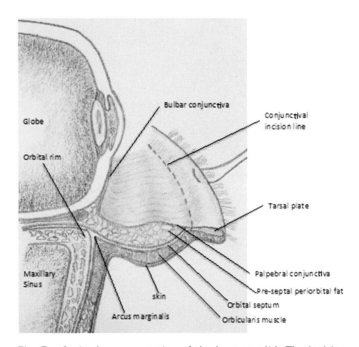

Fig. 7   Sagittal representation of the lower eyelid. The incision for the transconjunctival approach is represented by the dashed line inferior to the tarsal plate.

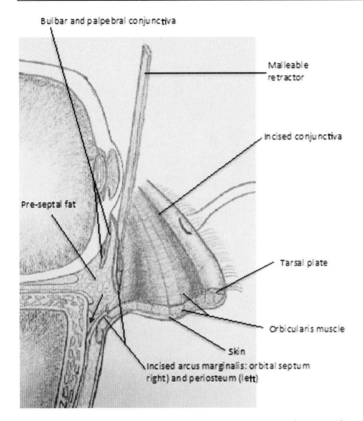

Bulbar and palpebral conjunctiva

Malleable retractor

Incised conjunctiva

Pre-septal fat

Tarsal plate

Orbicularis muscle

Skin

Incised arcus marginalis: orbital septum right) and periosteum (left)

Fig. 8 Sagittal representation of the transconjunctival approach for blepharoplasty. The preseptal dissection is completed bluntly with Metzenbaum scissors down to the orbital rim. Next, the arcus marginalis is incised, and the remainder of the dissection is completed in the subperiosteal plane, approximately 1 cm below the rim. This dissection is carried medially to include the tear trough deformity (not shown). Periorbital fat is then gently positioned in the base of the pocket.

suture is then passed twice through the tendon, in the same direction, with the needle left attached. Next, the LCT is secured to the periostium of the lateral orbital rim with the same nonresorbable suture. The authors advocate repositioning the LCT 2 mm higher than ideal to account for relapse. Closure is completed with interrupted 5-0 prolene for the skin, and the grey line is reapproximated with 6-0 fast.

Complications

In keeping with the conservative theme of the transconjunctival lower blepharoplasty, there are few complications unique to this procedure. As stated earlier, one of the major advantages of this approach is the decreased incidence of complications, namely, lid malposition, external scarring, canthal webbing, wound dehiscence, and most importantly, ectropion. However, as is the case with the transcutaneous

approach, the risk of the most serious complication, retrobulbar hematoma, is rare.

Discussion

With lower blepharoplasties, there is no secret to achieving successful results. As is the case with any surgical procedure, proper patient evaluation and development of a comprehensive, anatomic-based treatment plan are prerequisites for success. For situations in which a patient has little lid laxity and pseudoherniated periorbital fat, the transconjunctival lower blepharoplasty is the treatment of choice. This approach enables the surgeon to reposition fat, effectively blending the lid–cheek junction and filling the tear trough deformity.

In order to better enable clinicians to achieve optimal outcomes, the authors advocate an anatomic-based approach for patient evaluation and treatment planning. Application of this philosophy involves a well-founded understanding of lower eyelid anatomy and the pathophysiology of aging. With this essential knowledge, the surgeon will be best equipped for success.

References

1. Camirand A, Doucet J, Harris J. Anatomy, pathophysiology, and prevention of senile enopohtalmia and associated herniated lower eyelid fat pads. Plast Reconstr Surg 1997;100(6):1535–46.
2. Mendelson BC. Herniated fat and the orbital septum of the lower lid. Clin Plast Surg 1993;20:323.
3. Camirand A, Doucet J, Harris J. The aging eye: pathophysiology and management. Surg Technol Int 1997;5:347.
4. Doxanas MT, Anderson RL. Clinical orbital anatomy. Baltimore (MD): Williams & Wilkins; 1984.
5. Wolff E. The anatomy of the eye and orbit. Philadelphia: WB Saunders; 1976.
6. Zide BM. Surgical anatomy around the orbit: the system of zones. 2nd edition. Philadelphia: Lippincott, Williams & Wilkins; 2006.
7. Gioia VM, Linberg JV, McCormick S. The anatomy of the lateral canthal tendon. Arch Ophthalmol 1987;105(4):529–32.
8. Muzaffar AR, Mendelson BC, Adams WP Jr. Surgical anatomy of the ligamentous attachments of the lower lid and lateral canthus. Plast Reconstr Surg 2002;110(3):873–84.
9. Hill J. Analysis of senile changes in the palpebral fissure. Trans Ophthalmol Soc U K 1975;95:49.
10. Shore JW, McCord CD. Involutional changes in blepharoptosis. Ophthalmology 1984;98:21–7.
11. Raschke GF, Rieger UM, Bader RD, et al. Transconjunctival versus subciliary approach for orbital fracture repair—an anthropometric evaluation of 221 cases. Clin Oral Investig 2013;17(3):933–42.
12. Putterman AM. Scalpel neodymium:YAG laser in oculoplastic surgery. Am J Ophthalmol 1990;109:581–4.
13. Putterman AM. Treatment of conjunctival prolapse. Arch Ophthalmol 1995;113:553–4.
14. Goldberg RA. Transconjunctival orbital fat repositioning: transposition of orbital fat pedicles into a subperiosteal pocket. Plast Reconstr Surg 2000;105(2):743–8.

Management of Lower Eyelid Laxity

Gary Linkov, MD [a], Allan E. Wulc, MD [a,b,c,*]

KEYWORDS

• Lower eyelid laxity • Blepharoplasty complications • Canthal tightening • Lateral canthopexy • Lateral canthoplasty

KEY POINTS

• Lower eyelid laxity has various etiologies.
• In-office tests assess lower eyelid laxity and help to plan for correction at the time of lower blepharoplasty or to address postoperative lower blepharoplasty complications.
• Many surgical procedures to correct lower eyelid laxity do not address the canthus specifically or may be aggressive and should be reserved for complex reconstructive cases.
• The tarsal strip procedure is exceedingly valuable in patients who have severe laxity and simultaneous lower eyelid malposition, but is not ideal in the aesthetic patient.
• A modified canthal fixation procedure is proposed to address the shortcomings of other techniques and to offer an effective option with excellent long-term outcomes.

Introduction

Management of the lateral canthus is a vital consideration in lower blepharoplasty. Patients who exhibit preoperative laxity, canthal dystopia, or positive vertical vectors are all at risk to have complications with cosmetic lower blepharoplasty and may require modifications from standard technique to ensure aesthetic outcomes. The surgeon must be able to identify these at-risk patients. Similarly, the surgeon must be able to address the postoperative patient who develops lower eyelid ectropion or lateral canthal dystopia after lower blepharoplasty or midface lift.

This article reviews the anatomy of the lateral canthus. We describe the pathogenesis of lower eyelid and lateral canthal laxity, the preoperative assessment, and several procedures that can be used to address canthal laxity and dystopia in blepharoplasty. We also detail the management of the patient who presents with postblepharoplasty lower eyelid retraction.

Lateral canthal anatomy

The lateral canthus lies approximately 1 to 2 mm higher than the medial canthus, and in healthy adults is positioned less than

1 cm from the lateral orbital rim.[1] The horizontal palpebral fissure describes the distance between the medial and lateral commissures and ranges from 28 to 31 mm.[2] The lateral canthal angle is about 6° from a horizontal reference line[3] and measures about 60°.[2] The lateral canthus is a mobile structure: both the lateral horn of the levator aponeurosis, the lower eyelid retractors and the lateral rectus have attachments to the lateral canthal tendon (LCT), and as a result, movements of these anatomic components are translated to the canthus itself.

Unlike the medial canthal tendon, which has a tendinous portion in its anterior component that is anatomically demonstrable, the LCT is not visualized even during open surgery. An indistinct structure anatomically, it nonetheless has solid structural components that give rise to firm fibrous attachments to the lateral orbital rim in healthy patients. These fibrous attachments include the orbital septum, which corresponds to the anterior part of the LCT, and a posterior fibrous attachment to Whitnall's tubercle, a bony prominence approximately 1 cm within the orbit to which most lateral orbital supporting structures attach.[4]

The eyelids are conveniently divided into 3 lamellae: the anterior lamella (the skin and orbicularis oculi muscle), the middle lamella (the orbital septum and orbital fat), and the posterior lamella (the capsulopalpebral fascia and conjunctiva), and, at the lateral canthus, where the upper and lower eyelids meet, there are also 3 lamellae. Each of these lamellae needs to be addressed in reconstructive surgery of the canthus.

The orbicularis oculi muscle encircles the orbit and lies 4 to 6 mm below the dermis at the level of the brow, tapering to less than 0.1 mm at the pretarsal eyelid.[2] Extension of the orbicularis oculi muscle from the orbital rim has been found to be 14 mm superiorly, 12 mm inferiorly, and 25 mm laterally, all measured beyond the rim.[5] Fibrous septa emanate from the dermis and attach to the orbicularis muscle to form the anterior lamella. The orbicularis muscle is divided into pretarsal, preseptal, and orbital portions that envelop the corresponding portions of the eyelid.[2]

Funding: None.

Financial Disclosures: None.

Conflicts of Interest: None.

[a] Department of Otolaryngology — Head & Neck Surgery, Temple University School of Medicine, 3401 North Broad Street, Philadelphia, PA 19140, USA

[b] Department of Ophthalmology, Scheie Eye Institute, University of Pennsylvania, 51 North 39th Street, Philadelphia, PA 19104, USA

[c] Private Practice, W Cosmetic Surgery, 610 West Germantown Pike, Suite 161, Plymouth Meeting, PA 19462, USA

* Corresponding author. W Cosmetic Surgery, 610 West Germantown Pike, Suite 161, Plymouth Meeting, PA 19462.

E-mail address: awulcmd@gmail.com

http://dx.doi.org/10.1016/j.cxom.2016.05.009

The orbital septum in the lower eyelid has its origin at the arcus marginalis along the infraorbital rim and inserts into the capsulopalpebral fascia or lower eyelid retractors approximately 5 mm below the inferior tarsal border. It is a thin, fibrous layer in contiguity with the retroorbicularis fascia that contains the intraorbital fat compartment.[2] The capsulopalpebral fascia attaches to the inferior tarsal border and envelops the inferior oblique muscle, attaching to the lacrimal fascia and the anterior maxillary spine medially and the lateral canthus laterally.

The primary static support of the lower lid is the fibrous tarsocanthal complex. The tarsus in the lower lid measures approximately 3 to 4 mm in height (compared with 10 mm in the upper eyelid) and 20 mm in length, and is attached medially to the medial canthal tendon and laterally to Whitnall's tubercle.[6]

Secondary lid supports include the lower lid retractors, which help maintain the lid in anteroposterior balance, the orbicularis oculi muscle, which forms a muscular sling around the eyelid and orbital contents, and the globe itself, which prevents the eyelid from tilting posteriorly.[2]

The LCT originates from the lateral aspect of the tarsus, where it is contiguous with the lateral horn of the levator palpebrae aponeurosis. The length of LCT measured from canthal angle to insertion has been found to be 10 mm on average.[7] It inserts as a single limb on the medial aspect of the lateral orbital wall at Whitnall's tubercle, a region 1.5 to 2 mm posterior to the lateral orbital rim. The LCT is a component of the lateral retinaculum and fuses posteriorly with other structures including the check ligament of the lateral rectus muscle, the inferior suspensory ligament of Lockwood, the superior ligament of Whitnall, and the lateral horn of the levator aponeurosis. The posterior limb of the LCT is separated from its anterior component (contiguous with the orbital septum) anteriorly by fat within a compartment known as Eisler's pocket.[2]

Eisler's pocket is a fat-filled recess in the lateral lower eyelids, bounded by the orbital septum anteriorly and superiorly, the LCT posteriorly and nasally, the lateral orbital rim temporally, and the zygoma inferiorly.[8] It is clinically important because, to obtain posterior projection of the LCT in canthopexy, sutures must engage the fibrous tissue behind Eisler's pocket (the posterior limb of the LCT) and not the orbital septum alone.

Pathogenesis of eyelid laxity

Many of the changes that occur at the lateral canthus are involutional. Pessa and colleagues[9] have shown that the lower lateral orbit increases in vertical dimension with aging and that the vertical maxilla shortens and diminishes in projection, allowing the midface to shift inferiorly. This shift may cause the lower eyelid to bow laterally, and may allow the lower eyelid to drift medially and inferiorly with advancing age. Over time, traction on the lateral canthus may attenuate its attachments to the lower eyelid and may contribute to the laxity of the lower eyelid seen in older individuals. Bowing of the temporal lateral aspect of the lower eyelid can distract the lower eyelid from the surface of the globe, resulting in ectropion and in the potential for dry eye symptoms owing to increased exposure.

Cicatrical lower eyelid ectropion and round eye scleral show syndrome can result from aggressive anterior approach blepharoplasty or midface elevation procedures, from over-resection of skin, from middle lamella contracture, or from inadequate support of the lateral canthus in patients that are anatomically predisposed.

Certain conditions also predispose to canthal laxity. Floppy eyelid syndrome, the most common subtype of lax eyelid syndromes, is a condition that is seen with increased frequency in patients who are obese and who have sleep apnea. Floppy eyelid syndrome is more common in males, and has been described accompanying keratoconus[10] or hyperglycinemia.[11] Histologically, the tarsus is depleted of elastin adjacent to the lash follicles and the canthal tendons; therefore, both the medial and the lateral tendons are often lax or seem to be dehiscent.[12,13]

Paralysis of the lower eyelid, seen in facial palsies, can give rise to paralytic ectropion of the lid owing to orbicularis atony. Although the lateral canthus is not affected directly by paralytic ectropion, correction of the ectropion often involves manipulation of the lateral canthus.[2]

Assessment

A patient with canthal or lower eyelid laxity may exhibit dry eye symptoms, a foreign body sensation, or reflex tearing owing to eye irritation. However, the majority of patients will be asymptomatic and develop problems postoperatively. It is therefore important to identify the at-risk patient preoperatively.

The evaluation of the patient undergoing lower blepharoplasty routinely involves the assessment of vertical vectors. The patient who might develop eyelid retraction after blepharoplasty will have a relatively prominent eye as compared with the bony maxilla. Many of these predisposed patients have shallow bony orbits, axial myopia, or thyroid eye disease.

In these patients, the lower eyelid may be displaced anteriorly by the prominent eye. The sclera may be visible in primary gaze indicating lower eyelid scleral show. Patients of this sort are said to exhibit *negative vertical vectors*. A negative vector is present when the globe protrudes anterior to the inferior orbital rim (Fig. 1A, B). When a negative vector is present, the lid must support itself against the upward slope of the projection of the eye without bony orbital support. Lid tightening and/or skin excision in this situation may bowstring the lid under the globe and result in a worsening of eyelid position. A positive vector is the opposite situation, where the globe does not project beyond the midface, cheek or inferior orbital rim (Fig. 1C, D).[14]

Transconjunctival surgery, or conservative external blepharoplasty, should be considered as a preferred procedure in high-risk patients with a negative vector. Consideration should also be given to canthal suspension and eyelid support without attempts to tighten the lateral canthus in this group of patients, because an eyelid tightening may produce or exacerbate lower eyelid retraction.

An exophthalmometer is used routinely in our practice to identify and classify positive-negative vector patients. The degree of eye prominence is determined by the position of the globe relative to the bony orbit. Values of 13 to 15 mm using the Naugle-Hertel exophthalmometer are considered within the normal range, and values greater than this are often indicative of a negative vector.[15] Most types of exophthalmometer can provide similar diagnostic information.[16]

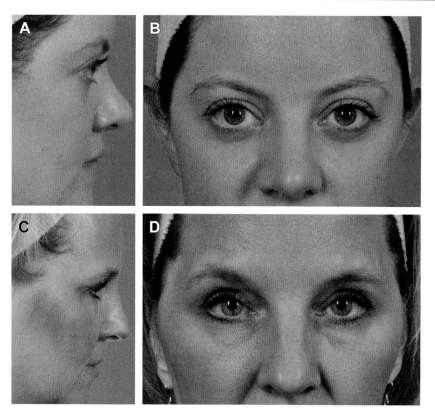

Fig. 1 Vectors. (*A*) Negative vector (lateral view): The globe protrudes anterior to the inferior orbital rim. (*B*) Negative vector (frontal view): Lower eyelids are displaced anteriorly by the prominent eyes. (*C*) Positive vector (lateral view): The globe does not project beyond the midface, cheek, or inferior orbital rim. (*D*) Positive vector (frontal view): Normal lower eyelid position is seen.

We routinely assess the prominent eye patient with exophthalmometry, evaluate old photographs to assess chronologic changes, and, when indicated, obtain thyroid studies and/or imaging if thyroid eye disease is suspected.

Palpation is exceedingly valuable in assessing canthal laxity. The lateral canthus should not be mobile—the surgeon should feel a firm stop when attempting to distract the LCT medially. Medial canthal laxity can be assessed with this technique as well. Mobility of the inferior punctum can be assessed as a measure of medial canthal laxity—one should not be able to distract the medial canthal tendon laterally by more than 5 mm. Medial canthal tendon laxity must also be treated if the lateral canthus is to be tightened. Otherwise, the punctum can be pulled erroneously laterally as far as the corneal limbus creating a noticeable deformity.

Eyelid and canthal laxity are also gauged with the snapback test by pulling the lower lid from the globe with the thumb and forefinger to check its ability to snap back to the globe. On release, the lid should return to its normal position immediately and certainly before the patient blinks (Fig. 2A, B).[17]

The lower eyelid distraction test involves pulling the lower eyelid away from the surface of the globe. If the eyelid can be pulled more than 6 to 10 mm from the cornea, the test result is abnormal (positive), which also indicates eyelid laxity (Fig. 2C).[18,19] An LCT tightening is indicated in patients with eyelid laxity determined by either of these latter tests.

In cases where lower blepharoplasty has already been performed, it is helpful to perform a lower eyelid forced duction—a test of the mobility of the lower eyelid. The patient is asked to look up while the examiner manually displaces the lower eyelid superiorly. Normally, the lower eyelid easily stretches upward to cover the entire cornea and close the eye. If the lower eyelid is mechanically restricted from moving upward, anterior or middle lamellar scarring is suspected.

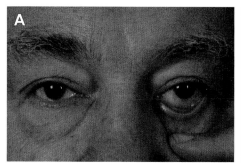 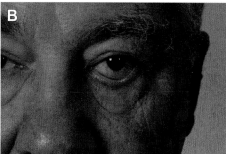 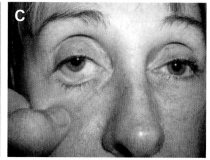

Fig. 2 In-office tests. (*A*) Snap back test: Lower lid is pulled away from the globe. (*B*) Snap back test: In this patient, the lid does not return to its normal position. (*C*) Distraction test: The lower lid is being pulled more than 6 to 10 mm from the cornea, indicating eyelid laxity.

In these cases, release of middle lamellar scarring, and, potentially, posterior lamellar spacer grafts or skin grafting may be required to restore eyelid position and allow for patient comfort and improved aesthetics.[18]

Procedures

Laterally based horizontal eyelid resection (bick)

This simple procedure is indicated in the patient that exhibits pure lower eyelid laxity and has firm canthal support. Originally described by Bick,[20] a triangle of full-thickness eyelid is excised and resutured at the canthal angle. It is a simple method of eyelid shortening that uses the firm attachments of the lower eyelid at the lateral canthus, but it does not actually address the canthus or alter its position. However, a hybrid procedure that combines features of the classic Bick procedure and lateral tarsal strip for correction of lower eyelid malpositions owing to horizontal laxity has previously been proposed.[21]

Tarsal Strip Procedure

Described by Anderson and Gordy in 1979,[22] the tarsal strip procedure addresses LCT laxity or malposition. It was designed to address cases of ectropion in which traditional lid shortening was inadequate.

After lateral canthotomy and cantholysis, an infraciliary incision is made. The lid is shortened conservatively, leaving a lateral area of redundancy that will provide support to the lateral canthus. A strip of tarsus is created by denuding the posterior tarsus of conjunctiva using a blade or a cautery, and trimming the lash follicles at their bases from the strip with a Westcott scissors. The tarsal strip is now sutured to the periosteum on the inner aspect of the lateral orbital wall and the lateral canthal angle is reformed with absorbable sutures.[23] Our refinement of this highly versatile procedure was described in 1991 (Figs. 3 and 6A).[24]

We have largely abandoned this procedure in aesthetic patients because it involves disruption of the supporting ligaments of the lateral orbit and may be unnecessary. Initial cutting of the tendon permits the lid to be mobilized excessively and tempts the surgeon to perform unduly large resections. The subsequent medial drift seen in these patients shortens the horizontal palpebral fissure and deprives the patient of their lower eyelid lashes. All too often we have encountered revision patients whose canthi and lower eyelids have been irreversibly distorted and who feel acutely the aesthetic consequences of the lash resection.

However, in the presence of severe lower eyelid and canthal laxity, a conservative tarsal strip may be helpful in restoring

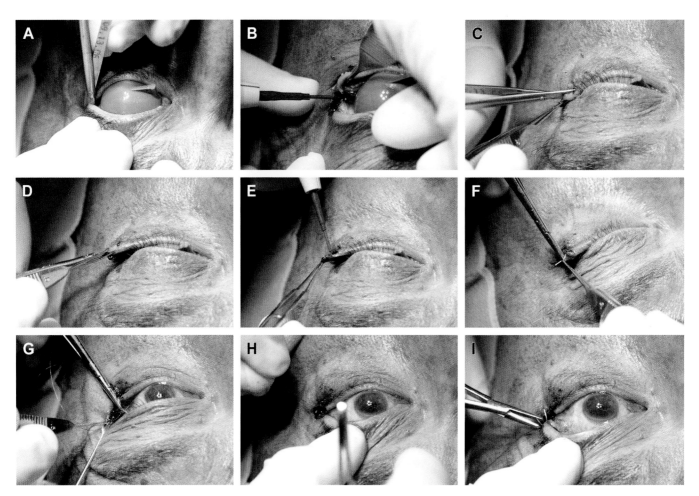

Fig. 3 Tarsal strip procedure. (*A*) Canthotomy. (*B*) Cantholysis. (*C*) Infraciliary incision. (*D*) Removal of lashes and amputation of lash segment. (*E*) Removal of upper mucocutaneous junction conjunctiva followed by denuding of the conjunctival surface. (*F*) Suture placed through the tarsus. (*G*) Suture needle placed through the orbital rim periosteum (*dashed line*). (*H*) Securing a double-armed suture to reform the lateral canthal angle. (*I*) Placing final suture through the gray line.

support to the lower eyelid and correcting ectropion and can be modified to treat entropion as well.

Simple canthal suspension

The canthus can be suspended by passing a double-armed suture through a button hole incision made at the lateral canthal angle and anchored to orbital periosteum after dividing the supporting ligaments. An external incision either lateral to the canthal angle or in the upper lid allows the supporting ligaments of the LCT to be divided and the anchoring double-armed suture position can be visualized as it engages orbital periosteum. Placement of this double-armed suture provides a powerful means of altering the vertical placement of the canthus as well as of augmenting horizontal fissure length. It allows the canthus to be placed in a variety of positions, supraplaced or infraplaced. As such, it is important to verify symmetry when performing this surgery (Fig. 4).[14,25]

Lateral canthal anchoring

In the complex patient, the canthus can be fixated using a wire technique, passing stainless steel wire through the zygomatic bone. However, we have found that failure of canthal support occurs not owing to loss of bony suspension, but rather to loss of soft tissue fixation. This occurs regardless of whether wire or suture is used to obtain purchase to bone or soft tissue. We have therefore abandoned this technique. However, other authors find it helpful.[26]

Modified canthal fixation procedure

Our preferred canthal suspension technique accompanies many of our lower eyelid cosmetic blepharoplasty in the predisposed patient and involves a noncutting canthal tightening procedure. It is performed in conjunction with lower

blepharoplasty, facilitating the transconjunctival procedure by relaxing the lateral canthus. It allows the surgeon to suspend the canthus in the desired position and attains long-lasting results with minimal dissection and canthal disruption.

Description of procedure
Tetracaine drops are instilled into the eyes. After infiltrating the eyelid and the lateral canthus with local anesthetic including adrenaline, using a 30-gauge needle, the patient is prepped and draped in the usual sterile manner. An approximately 4.5-mm incision is made at the lateral canthus, sparing the lateral canthal angle, approximately 2 mm lateral to the lateral canthal angle. The incision can be varied and an upper eyelid crease incision can be used for this procedure if a concomitant upper blepharoplasty is performed. Alternatively, if a skin pinch is to be removed, the incision can be lowered 2 to 3 mm below the lateral canthus and extended in an infraciliary fashion across the lower eyelid to avoid a lateral dog ear.

Dissection is carried below the orbicularis. Grasping the lateral edge of the inferior lid with a 0.5-mm forceps, the eyelid is suspended using a 4-0 Vicryl (Ethicon, Somerville, NJ) on a half circular P-2 needle, passing the suture partial thickness through the inferior tarsus at the edge of the lateral canthus. The suture is now deployed deep to the orbital rim along the posterior lateral wall of the orbit at the desired canthal location. This suture is passed in an attempt to engage the posterior portion of the LCT adjacent to Whitnall's tubercle. A second cleft palate needle is now used to create a double-armed horizontal mattress suture, also placing the suture through the posterior portion of the LCT. The pathway of both sutures determines the desired height and position of the lateral canthus.

Before securing the suture, the analogous procedure is performed on the contralateral side and the desired position of the canthus and its symmetry is ensured. The skin is now closed with interrupted sutures per the surgeon's preference (Figs. 5 and 6B).

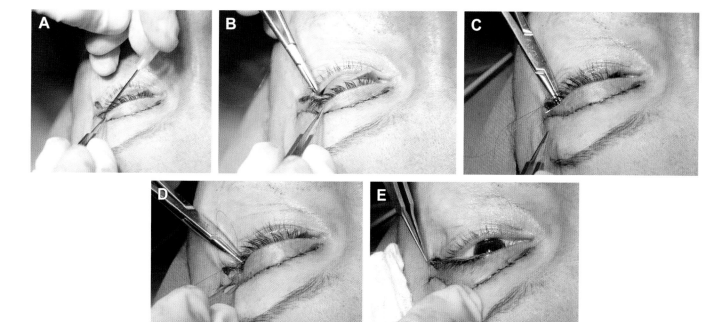

Fig. 4 Simple canthal suspension. (*A*) Sharp needle used to create a buttonhole incision in the lateral canthus. (*B*) External incision lateral to the canthal angle. Suture needle about to engage the lateral canthus. (*C*) Needle trajectory (*dashed line*) of the anchoring double-armed suture. (*D*) Suture position visualized as it engages orbital periosteum. (*E*) Repositioned lateral canthus.

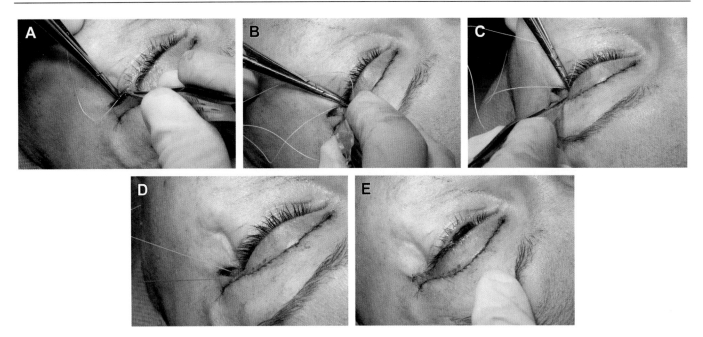

Fig. 5 Modified canthal fixation procedure. (*A*) Grasping the lateral edge of the inferior lid with a 0.5-mm forceps, the eyelid is suspended using a 4-0 Vicryl on a half circular P-2 needle, passing the suture partial thickness through the inferior tarsus at the edge of the lateral canthus (*dashed line*). (*B, C*) The suture is deployed deep to the orbital rim along the posterior lateral wall of the orbit at the desired canthal location. (*D*) A second cleft palate needle is used to create a double-armed horizontal mattress suture with both sutures suspended, the upper and lower, at the desired height of the lateral canthus. (*E*) Lateral incision closed with 6-0 fast-absorbing gut suture.

Adjunctive procedures

If a patient presents with postoperative lower eyelid mid-lamellar or canthal dystopia after blepharoplasty, adjunctive procedures may need to be performed to supplement over-resection of fat or skin, or contraction of the middle lamella. Midlamellar deficiencies are addressed with hard palate mucosa or dermis–fat interpositional grafting to the middle lamella of the lower eyelid. Overresection of fat can be treated with liposculpture, and midfacial soft tissue can be recruited using a variety of midface elevation techniques to diminish the need for full-thickness skin grafting. Most of these procedures involve simultaneous tightening or repositioning of the lateral canthus using the techniques described elsewhere in this article.

Complications

Conservative canthal surgery should not give rise to severe complications. However, procedures such as wire fixation and the tarsal strip procedure can disrupt the canthus and cause decreased orbicularis function, lash loss, and scarring. Overtightening of the lateral canthus can result in lid imbrication syndrome, where the loose upper eyelid overrides the tightened lower eyelid with lid closure.[27] Medial drift of the lateral canthus can occur after degloving of preexisting attachments at the lateral canthus.[14]

Commonly observed complications with the technique we describe for lower blepharoplasty with canthal tightening include granulomas at the incision site from the absorbable sutures, and, rarely, dehiscence owing to suture failure. In

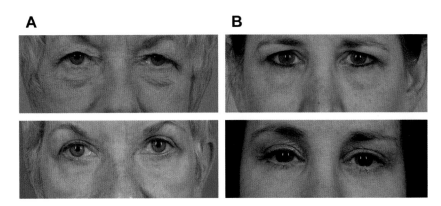

Fig. 6 Patient outcomes. (*A*) Before the tarsal strip procedure (*top image*) and after the tarsal strip procedure (*bottom image*). Procedure combined with upper and lower blepharoplasty. (*B*) Before the modified canthal fixation procedure (*top image*) and after the modified canthal fixation procedure (*bottom image*). Procedure combined with upper and lower blepharoplasty.

cases of dehiscence, or poor placement of the fixation sutures, revisional surgery may be required.

Summary

- Lower eyelid laxity has various etiologies. In-office tests are used to assess lower eyelid laxity and to plan for correction at the time of lower blepharoplasty or to address postoperative lower blepharoplasty complications.
- Many surgical procedures to correct lower eyelid laxity do not address the canthus specifically or may be aggressive with the potential for untoward aesthetic consequences and should be reserved for complex reconstructive cases.
- The tarsal strip procedure is exceedingly valuable in patients who have severe laxity and simultaneous lower eyelid malposition, but is not ideal in the aesthetic patient.
- A modified canthal fixation procedure, often accompanying a lower cosmetic blepharoplasty, is proposed to address the shortcomings of other techniques and to offer an effective option with excellent long-term outcomes.

References

1. Chong KK, Goldberg RA. Lateral canthal surgery. Facial Plast Surg 2010;26(3):193—200.
2. Bergeron CM, Moe KS. The evaluation and treatment of lower eyelid paralysis. Facial Plast Surg 2008;24(2):231—41.
3. Vasanthakumar P, Kumar P, Rao M. Anthropometric analysis of palpebral fissure dimensions and its position in South Indian ethnic adults. Oman Med J 2013;28(1):26—32.
4. Whitnall SE. The anatomy of the human orbit and accessory organs of vision. London: Frowde and Hodder & Stoughton; 1921.
5. Costin BR, Sakolsatayadorn N, McNutt SA, et al. Dimensions and anatomic variations of the orbicularis oculi muscle in non-preserved, fresh-frozen human cadavers. Ophthal Plast Reconstr Surg 2014;30(2):198—200.
6. De Silva DJ, Prasad A. Aesthetic canthal suspension. Clin Plast Surg 2015;42(1):79—86.
7. Gioia VM, Linberg JV, McCormick SA. The anatomy of the lateral canthal tendon. Arch Ophthalmol 1987;105(4):529—32.
8. Bartley GB, Gerber TC. Eisler and his pocket. Am J Ophthalmol 2006;141(2):417—8.
9. Pessa JE, Desvigne LD, Lambros VS, et al. Changes in ocular globe-to-orbital rim position with age: implications for aesthetic blepharoplasty of the lower eyelids. Aesthetic Plast Surg 1999; 23(5):337—42.
10. Donnenfeld ED, Perry HD, Gibralter RP, et al. Keratoconus associated with floppy eyelid syndrome. Ophthalmology 1991;98(11): 1674—8.
11. Gerner EW, Hughes SM. Floppy eyelid with hyperglycinemia. Am J Ophthalmol 1984;98(5):614—6.
12. Belliveau MJ, Harvey JT. Floppy eyelid syndrome. CMAJ 2015; 187(2):130.
13. Fowler AM, Dutton JJ. Floppy eyelid syndrome as a subset of lax eyelid conditions: relationships and clinical relevance (an ASOPRS thesis). Ophthal Plast Reconstr Surg 2010;26(3):195—204.
14. Massry GG. Comprehensive lower eyelid rejuvenation. Facial Plast Surg 2010;26(3):209—21.
15. Cole HP 3rd, Couvillion JT, Fink AJ, et al. Exophthalmometry: a comparative study of the Naugle and Hertel instruments. Ophthal Plast Reconstr Surg 1997;13(3):189—94.
16. Hirmand H, Codner MA, McCord CD, et al. Prominent eye: operative management in lower lid and midfacial rejuvenation and the morphologic classification system. Plast Reconstr Surg 2002;110(2): 620—8 [discussion: 629—34].
17. McGraw BL, Adamson PA. Postblepharoplasty ectropion. Prevention and management. Arch Otolaryngol Head Neck Surg 1991; 117(8):852—6.
18. Griffin G, Azizzadeh B, Massry GG. New insights into physical findings associated with postblepharoplasty lower eyelid retraction. Aesthet Surg J 2014;34(7):995—1004.
19. Jindal K, Sarcia M, Codner MA. Functional considerations in aesthetic eyelid surgery. Plast Reconstr Surg 2014;134(6): 1154—70.
20. Bick MW. Surgical management of orbital tarsal disparity. Arch Ophthalmol 1966;75(3):386—9.
21. Barrett RV, Meyer DR. The modified Bick quick strip procedure for surgical treatment of eyelid malposition. Ophthal Plast Reconstr Surg 2012;28(4):294—9.
22. Anderson RL, Gordy DD. The tarsal strip procedure. Arch Ophthalmol 1979;97(11):2192—6.
23. Della Rocca DA. The lateral tarsal strip: illustrated pearls. Facial Plast Surg 2007;23(3):200—2.
24. Weber PJ, Popp JC, Wulc AE. Simultaneous lateral, anterior, and posterior (SLAP) lower-lid blepharoplasty. Ophthalmic Surg 1992; 23(4):260—4.
25. Georgescu D, Anderson RL, McCann JD. Lateral canthal resuspension sine canthotomy. Ophthal Plast Reconstr Surg 2011;27(5): 371—5.
26. McCord CD, Ford DT, Hanna K, et al. Lateral canthal anchoring: special situations. Plast Reconstr Surg 2005;116(4):1149—57.
27. Donnenfeld ED, Perry HD, Schrier A, et al. Lid imbrication syndrome. Diagnosis with rose Bengal staining. Ophthalmology 1994; 101(4):763—6.

Open Brow Lift Surgery for Facial Rejuvenation

Tirbod Fattahi, MD, DDS

KEYWORDS

• Brow lift • Forehead lift • Pretrichial brow lift

KEY POINTS

• Brow lifting is a gratifying operation; creation of a youthful eye/brow complex can by quite dramatic.
• Repositioning of the brows can aid in the appearance of other structures of the upper face, such as the forehead rhytids, glabellar muscles, crow's feet, and upper eye lids.
• Although there are several acceptable methods of brow elevation, a pretrichial brow lift is a predictable, stable, and simple operation to satisfy the cosmetic needs of patients.

Introduction

Brow lifting has been around in the surgical armamentarium for nearly 100 years. Passot in 1919 first described using transverse skin excision of upper forehead skin to elevate the brows.[1] In 1926, Hunt described coronal and hairline excision to achieve a similar result.[2] In the following years, undermining of the pericranium and resection of corrugator muscles became popular.[3] In the 1960s, other modifications such as the pretrichial incision were introduced.[4] In the 1970s, the first description of a "biplanar" approach to the temporal region was described.[5] Flowers has been given credit for emphasizing the importance of establishment of proper brow positioning before upper eye lid surgery.[6] In 1992, Isse introduced the concept of minimally invasive forehead lifting via the endoscopic approach.[7] Since then, there have been a number of modifications to both the "open" and "endoscopic" approaches for brow lifting.[8–18]

This article describes the pretrichial brow lifting. Other types of forehead rejuvenation are described in another article (see Jon D. Perenack's article, "The Endoscopic Brow Lift," in this issue).

Indication for brow lift

Brow lifting is essentially synonymous with *forehead lifting*; the terms are used interchangeably throughout this article. Irrespective of the type of forehead lifting, the main indication for any type of forehead lifting is to create a more youthful position for brows. Repositioning of the brows to a more appropriate position can also aid in the appearance of other structures of the upper face such as softening of the forehead rhytids, relaxation of glabellar muscles (corrugator, procerous, and depressor supercilia), improvement in appearance of

crow's feet, and enhancing the appearance of upper eye lids (by improving dermatochalasia of upper lids). An open, bright, and youthful appearance of the eyes and brows, especially in a female, is often one of the first facial features noticed by most people. Patients who have upper eye lid dermatochalasia or fullness often have concomitant brow ptosis. In fact, placing the brows to their proper position in many cases resolves the upper lid fullness.

Advantages of pretrichial brow lift

Pretrichial brow lifting falls in the category of open brow lifting. Other popular open brow lifting techniques include the coronal brow lift as well as mid forehead and direct brow lifting. Endoscopic brow lifting is the other popular technique utilized by many and is discussed in another article (see Jon D. Perenack's article, "The Endoscopic Brow Lift," in this issue).

Ultimately, regardless of the specific approach of brow lifting, elevation of the forehead and rejuvenation of the brows are the only objectives. Clinicians often argue over "inherent" advantages of one cosmetic procedure over another based on anecdotal or "personal" preference and experience. Although one should never argue against experience and consistency of a particular technique, there are a few advantages of the pretrichial brow lifting over other methods. These include:

• Can allow shortening of a long forehead if necessary.
• Can bring anterior hair line more anteriorly if desired.
• No need for special equipment (endoscopic tower and/or instruments).
• No need for fixation devices (resorbable anchors, etc).

Patient selection

Ideal patient for the pretrichial brow lifting is any patient with brow ptosis with normal or elongated forehead. Patient's hair style must be taken into consideration because the incision is placed just inside the hair-bearing scalp. Patients who wear

Author has no financial disclosures or external sources of funding.

Department of Oral &Maxillofacial Surgery, University of Florida, 653-1 West 8th Street, 2nd Floor LRC Building, Jacksonville, FL 32209, USA

E-mail address: Tirbod.Fattahi@Jax.Ufl.Edu

http://dx.doi.org/10.1016/j.cxom.2016.05.003
oralmaxsurgeryatlas.theclinics.com

their hair combed or pulled back, as opposed to having bangs, must be counseled appropriately because the incision may be perceptible for a few weeks after surgery. As mentioned, brow lifting, regardless of the technique, should always precede upper eye lid blepharoplasty. Evaluation of forehead rhytids, both dynamic and static, in transverse and vertical fashion must also be accounted for (Fig. 1). Good quality preoperative photography is a must, as is in all cosmetic procedures. Forehead skin must also be evaluated; patients with rosacea or oily sebaceous skin tend to have "thick" and "heavy" forehead skin. It is the opinion and observation of the author that patients with thicker forehead skin may have a higher tendency for relapse if appropriate elevation and release of the forehead flap has not occurred. Assessment of the forehead length is also important; pretrichial brow lifting can reduce an excessively long forehead and it can also bring a receding hairline anteriorly. Also, measurement of the actual brow ptosis (comparing the position of the brows with the underlying supraorbital rim) is important, as is recognition of brow asymmetry. Significant brow asymmetry occurs quite frequently.

Surgical technique

Pretrichial brow lifting can be performed under sedation or under general anesthesia. The patient should be placed in a supine position in a reverse Trendelenburg position to elevate the head. A single dose of perioperative antibiotic is administered. After appropriate skin preparation, hair should be combed posteriorly to reveal the anterior hair line. One often can see fine vellus type of hair just anterior to the formal hairline. An extremely irregular incision is marked a few millimeters inside the hairline between the 2 temporal fusion lines (Fig. 2). The irregularity of this incision is important to aid in camouflaging the scar in the future. Local anesthetic with a vasoconstrictor is then injected for hemostasis. After waiting for the vasoconstrictive effects to begin to work, an anteriorly beveled incision is made. The bevel is critical in preserving as many hair follicles as possible on the hair-bearing scalp side of the incision (Fig. 3). If properly performed, hair growth will appear in and around the final incision within 3 to 4 months from these preserved follicles. The elevation of the flap is done in the subgaleal plane; others have advocated elevation in a subcutaneous plane.[15–17] It is

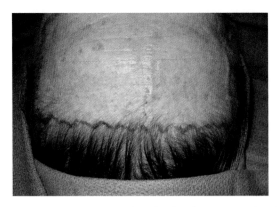

Fig. 2   Irregular incision within the hairline. Note the dotted lines along the temporal fusion lines.

the opinion and observation of the author that a subgaleal plane is easier, just as effective as a subcutaneous elevation, and, most important, augments the vascularity of the forehead flap.[18] Subgaleal elevation also protects the frontal branches of the facial nerve that travel in the subtemoporparietal fascia just above the galea. Elevation of the flap is performed bluntly all the way inferiorly beyond the brows. Because the elevation is in the subgaleal plane, there is no need to release the arcus marginalis, although this can be accomplished if necessary across the frontal bar. The forehead flap is essentially an axially based flap based on the supraorbital and supratrochlear arteries. The lateral aspects of this forehead flap are the temporal fusion lines; in cases where significant brow ptosis is present, especially laterally, release of the temporal fusion lines might be necessary to enhance flap elevation.

Once the flap is properly elevated, there should be a significant amount of overlap of the forehead flap and the intact

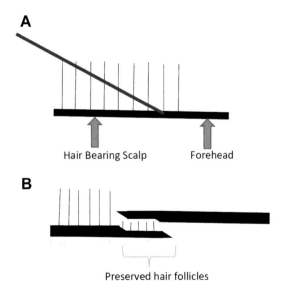

Fig. 3   Extreme bevel (*red line, A*) to preserve as many hair follicles on the hair-bearing scalp as possible (*B*). This will ensure future hair growth anterior to incision.

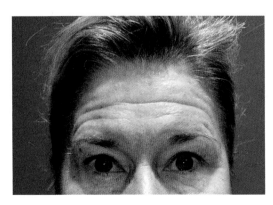

Fig. 1   Note static rhytids of forehead, brow ptosis, and fullness of upper eyelids.

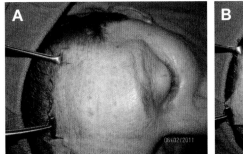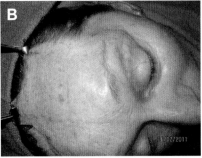

Fig. 4 (*A*, *B*) Note level of elevation and overlap of the forehead flap on the left side.

hair-bearing scalp (Fig. 4). If the hair-bearing scalp needs to be mobilized anteriorly, it is also undermined in a subgaleal plane and advanced anteriorly. Once satisfied with new position of the brows, the forehead flap is divided in the middle via a short vertical back-cut. This allows creation of a right and left flap; insetting of individual flap is easier than having to work with the entire forehead flap. Next surgical staples are placed to keep the forehead flap in its elevated state. Finally, the excess skin off the forehead flap is trimmed away; it is important to create a matching irregular pattern on the excision to match the initial irregular incision on the hair-bearing side. This type of excision maintains the overall length of the forehead; if necessary, elevate the hair-bearing scalp and move it anteriorly and then remove the excess forehead skin. This allows the anterior hair line to move anteriorly and shorten the forehead.

Closure is performed in layers using long-lasting, resorbable sutures for the deep side. Fibrin sealant are an excellent idea before closure of the deep surface. Fibrin sealants can act as a "belt and suspenders" by adding more stability to the new position of the elevated forehead flap. Skin closure is typically performed with resorbable sutures.

After surgery, hair is gently washed and dried in the operating room. A pressure dressing is then placed, which remains in place until the patient is seen in in 24 hours.

Postoperative care

The patient is seen within 24 hours after surgery to rule out any hematoma or seroma formation. Dressing can be re-applied for a few more days. Patients are instructed to keep their head dry for 48 hours, after which they can begin to shower. Postoperative hypoesthesia of the forehead is typical and can last for a few weeks. Final photographs are taken in about 3 to 4 months after surgery (Fig. 5).

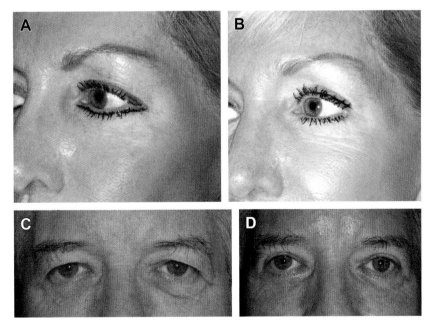

Fig. 5 (*A–D*) Before and after photos follow pretrichial brow lift.

Summary

Brow lifting is a gratifying operation. Creation of a youthful eye/brow complex can by quite dramatic. Although there are several acceptable methods of brow elevation, a pretrichial brow lift is a predictable, stable, and simple operation to satisfy the cosmetic needs of patients.

References

1. Passot R. Chirurgie Esthetique des rides du visage. Presse Med 1919;27:258.
2. Hunt HL. Plastic surgery of the head, face and neck. Philadelphia: Lea and Febiger; 1926.
3. Fomon S. Surgery of injury and plastic repair. Baltimore (MD): Williams and Wilkins; 1939.
4. Marino H, Gandolfo E. Treatment of forehead wrinkles. Prensa Med Argent 1964;34:406.
5. Regnault P. Complete face and forehead lifting, with double traction on crow's feet. Plast Reconstr Surg 1972;49:123.
6. Flowers RS. Periorbital aesthetic surgery for men: eyelids and related structures. Clin Plast Surg 1991;18:689.
7. Isse NG. Endoscopic facial rejuvenation: endoforehead, the functional lift. Case reports. Aesthetic Plast Surg 1994;18:21–9.
8. Perkins SW, Batniji RK. Trichophytic endoscopic forehead-lifting in high hairline patients. Facial Plast Surg Clin North Am 2006;14:185–93.
9. Vinas J, Caviglia C, Cortinas JL. Forehead rhytidoplasty and brow lifting. Plast Reconstr Surg 1976;57:445.
10. Ramirez OM. Anchor subperiosteal forehead lift: from open to endoscopic. Plast Reconstr Surg 2001;107:868.
11. Niamtu J. Endoscopic brow and forehead lift: a case for new technology. J Oral Maxillofac Surg 2006;64:1464.
12. Rowe DJ, Guyuron B. Optimizing results in endoscopic forehead rejuvenation. Clin Plast Surg 2008;35:355.
13. Nahai FR. The varied options in brow lifting. Clin Plast Surg 2013;40:101.
14. Javidnia H, Sykes J. Endoscopic brow lifts: have they replaced coronal lifts? Facial Plast Surg Clin North Am 2013;21:191.
15. Owsley TG. Subcutaneous trichophytic forehead browlift: the case for an open approach. J Oral Maxillofac Surg 2006;64:1133–6.
16. Guyuron B, Davies B. Subcutaneous anterior hairline forehead rhytidectomy. Aesthetic Plast Surg 1988;12:77–83.
17. Holcomb JD, McCollough EG. Trichophytic incisional approaches to upper facial rejuvenation. Arch Facial Plast Surg 2001;3:48–53.
18. Fattahi T. Trichophytic brow lift: a modification. Int J Oral Maxillofac Surg 2015;44:371–3.

The Endoscopic Brow Lift

Jon D. Perenack, MD, DDS [a,b,*]

KEYWORDS

- Endoscopic brow lift • Brow ptosis • Forehead rejuvenation • Brow-lift fixation • Brow asymmetry correction

KEY POINTS

- The endoscopic brow lift is most ideally suited to the patient exhibiting brow ptosis, redundant forehead/temporal skin, and a normal to short hairline.
- Specialized instruments are required to perform an endoscopic brow lift.
- Preoperative marking is designed to elevate the maximal arch of the brow superiorly and slightly medially. The temporal flap is elevated posterior superiorly along a vector from ala to lateral canthus.
- The endoscope is only used to visualize the dissection of the supraorbital and zygomaticotemporal bundles, and the periosteal release and any modifications of the muscles of facial expression.
- Most long-term complications of the endoscopic brow-lift procedure are related to inadequate periosteal release and fixation or utilization of improper vectors of pull and aggressive myotomy.

Brow lift general considerations

Various brow-lifting techniques have been described that can be used to modify the upper facial third. The endoscopic brow-lift procedure primarily provides the ability to elevate the brows and flatten forehead/temporal skin that is ptotic and redundant. Secondarily, correction of minor asymmetries in brow height, modification of the muscles of upper facial expression, and elevation of the hairline with elongation of the upper facial third can also be accomplished to some degree if desired. Although these same modifications can be achieved with either a coronal or a trichophytic brow-lift technique, the endoscopic approach has the advantage of smaller incision and scar load and improved patient acceptance.

Indications

Browptosis, secondary to aging, trauma, congenital deformity
Pseudo blepharoptosis, secondary to brow ptosis
Brow height and shape asymmetry
Redundant forehead skin with deep rhytids and furrows in the glabella/nasal radix, and the horizontal plane of the forehead
Short forehead/upper facial third

Disclosures: None.
[a] LSU Department of Oral and Maxillofacial Surgery, New Orleans, LA, USA
[b] Williamson Cosmetic Surgery Center, 8150 Jefferson Highway, Baton Rouge, LA 70809, USA
* Williamson Cosmetic Surgery Center, 8150 Jefferson Highway, Baton Rouge, LA 70809.
E-mail addresses: drperenack@cosmeticbr.com; jperen@hotmail.com

Contraindications

Lagophthalmos: incompetent lid seal at rest.

Relative contraindications

High forehead/elongated upper facial third
Concurrent upper blepharoplasty
History of symptomatic dry eyes accompanied by incompetent lid seal with simulated brow lift
Need for bony supra orbital rim recontouring

Evaluation and diagnosis

Evaluation of the potential endoscopic brow-lift patient should include a history and physical examination with particular emphasis on any history of dry eye symptoms or ocular disturbances such as lid ptosis, canthal laxity, and visual field defects. Patients who present with complaints of upper eyelid heaviness but also suffer from dry eye or lid seal abnormalities, and have concurrent brow ptosis, often tolerate a brow lift better to alleviate their cosmetic concerns than an upper blepharoplasty.[1]

Brow ptosis

The physical diagnosis of brow ptosis is made based on the position of the inferior aspect of the brow to the supraorbital rim. Male and female normative values for brow height should be considered (Fig. 1), but often it is just as useful to have the patient look in a full face mirror and manually simulate the potential brow elevation.[2,3] Some patients may prefer a high arching brow, while others may not like the appearance of having their brow elevated much past the supraorbital rim.

Atlas Oral Maxillofacial Surg Clin N Am 24 (2016) 165-173
1061-3315/16/$ - see front matter © 2016 Elsevier Inc. All rights reserved.
http://dx.doi.org/10.1016/j.cxom.2016.05.005

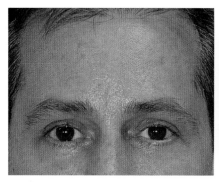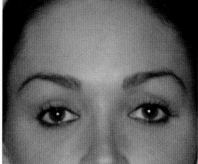

Fig. 1 Preoperative measurements guide treatment planning. Male brow describes an arc that typically follows at or 0 to 2 mm above the supraorbital rim with uniform upper-lid-to-brow distance; women display variable lid-to-brow distance with a lateral arch that may be 10 mm above the rim.

Brow-lifting simulation allows the surgeon to assess what the patient's internal goals for the surgery might be and if they are achievable. In addition, brow-lift simulation aids in determining if the patient is best served by a brow lift versus upper blepharoplasty, versus combined/staged brow lift and upper blepharoplasty. In patients with dry eye and lid seal abnormalities, the simulated brow lift allows the surgeon to assess if the planned brow lift will create lagophthalmos that would not be tolerated. The interbrow distance, brow shape and asymmetries, and degree of plucking should also be noted.

Forehead/temporal redundancy

Forehead, glabellar, and temporal skin redundancy and rhytids should also be assessed. Patients with heavy redundancy often see remarkable rejuvenation of the forehead after brow lift in this regard. It is important to distinguish true upper lid dermatochalasis from pseudo dermatochalasis, or as is often seen, assess the degree of the presence of both diagnoses. Prominent pseudo dermatochalasis often is associated with a visual field defect in the upper outer quadrant. If documentation of this is required for insurance purposes, referral to an optometrist is recommended. If residual upper lid dermatochalasis is noted with a simulated brow lift, it is important to discuss this with the patient and consider a concurrent or staged upper blepharoplasty if optimal correction is desired.

Hairline

The patient's hairline relative to their vertical facial thirds should be assessed along with any evidence of male- or female-pattern hair loss. As the endoscopic technique for brow lifting tends to visually elongate the upper facial third, any patient with a high hairline that is considering a brow lift should be offered a trichophytic hairline-lowering approach as an option.

Cosmetic botulinum toxin therapy

The patient should also be asked if they use cosmetic botulinum toxin therapy for the upper facial third. These patients often are not able to elevate their brows and may complain of brow heaviness. Although there are endoscopic techniques for reducing muscle hyperactivity via myotomies, the author always recommends to the patient that a brow lift may reduce the need for botulinum toxin therapy, but that it is

often still helpful in the period after brow lift. For the non-botulinum-toxin–treated patient, the degree of hyperactivity of the frontalis, corrugators/procerus, and orbicularis oculi should be assessed. In patients that exhibit a strong depressor habit (scowling, frowning, and squinting), the author recommends botulinum toxin therapy to reduce muscle activity. Optimally, this is performed at least 7 days before surgery.[4,5]

Skin

The surgeon should also assess for the presence of rhytids in the relaxed forehead/temple. The Glogau wrinkle score is a useful scale, but many other wrinkle scoring techniques have also been described. The patient should be aware that fine rhytids are best treated with a skin resurfacing or dermal tightening modality.

Evaluation key points

1. The endoscopic brow lift is most ideally suited to the patient exhibiting brow ptosis, redundant forehead/temporal skin, and a normal to short hairline.
2. Brow-lift simulation allows the patient and surgeon to better communicate about desired results and the possible need for upper eyelid surgery.
3. Textural and fine rhytid changes in the forehead skin are best treated with other modalities.

Clinical technique

Armamentarium

The endoscopic brow-lifting technique requires a special armamentarium that is not required for most open approaches: specifically, a 5-mm 30° rigid endoscope with retractor/cowling and a variety of curved endoscopic dissectors, scissors, and electrocautery (Fig. 2). The surgeon must also consider what fixation method should be used to produce a predictable result not prone to relapse. Multiple options exist, including suture fixation to screws, plates, and bone tunnels. Resorbable fixation devices are also available that engage both the periosteum and the underlying bone.[1]

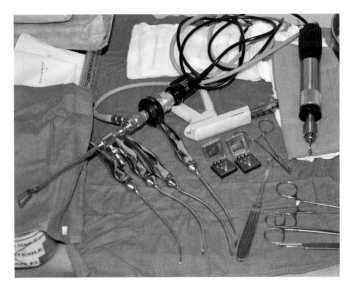

Fig. 2   Endoscopic instruments, 30° endoscope, Endotine setup.

Preoperative technique

1. The patient is marked in an upright, seated position with no facial animation after preoperative photos have been procured (Fig. 3). The supraorbital notch and proposed highest point of brow arch are marked. Three incisions are generally planned for the fontal hairline, 1 median and 2 paramedian. These incisions are usually placed 5 to 10 mm posterior to the hairline and are 2 cm in length. An attempt is made to avoid the natural part of the patient's hair. The paramedian incisions are marked vertically above and slightly medial to the planned highest point of the brow arch (Fig. 4).

2. Two temporal incisions are marked parallel to and posterior to the temporal hairline. The temporal incisions are typically 3 cm in length and are centered on a vector line drawn from ala through lateral canthus extended into the hairline. No shaving of the incision sites is recommended.

Anesthesia technique

1. Local anesthesia infiltration along supraorbital and lateral orbital rims
2. Tumescent solution injected subperiosteally from the supraorbital rim to slightly posterior to the vertex between the superior temporal lines
3. Tumescent solution injected bilaterally to fill the superficial temporal spaces
4. General anesthesia versus intravenous (IV)/intramuscular sedation techniques: although the endoscopic brow-lift procedure can be accomplished with local and tumescent anesthesia alone, for patient comfort, it is advisable to consider a general anesthesia or IV sedation technique (Fig. 5).

Operative technique

1. The patient is placed in a supine position on the operating room table, and appropriate monitors and alarms are used based on the anesthesia technique.
2. Corneal shields are preferable to lubricating and taping the eyes if a general anesthesia technique is selected.
3. The face and hair are prepared with a chlorhexidine solution, and the patient is sterilely draped to expose from vertex to the chin.
4. A No. 15 blade is used to carry the median and paramedian incisions down to bone. A No. 9 periosteal elevation begins the subperiosteal dissection, and a curved endoscopic

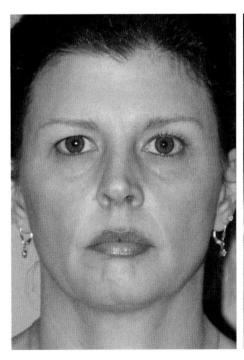
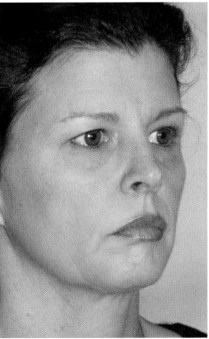
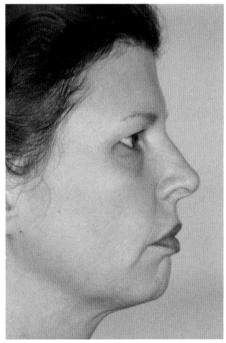

Fig. 3   Preoperative photos for endoscopic brow lift.

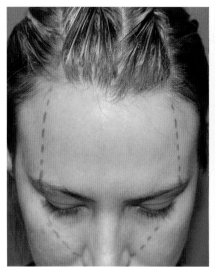 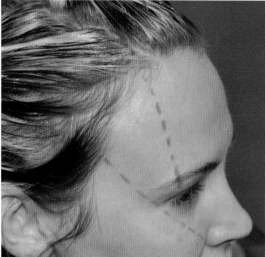 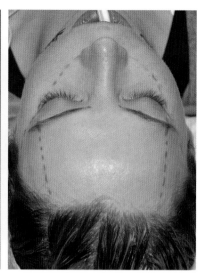

Fig. 4   Planned incision sites.

periosteal elevator is used to elevate the skin/soft tissue envelope subperiosteally from 2 cm above the supraorbital rim to the vertex. Laterally, this dissection is carried to the insertion point of the superficial temporoparietal fascia in the superior temporal line (Fig. 6).

5. A small 4-mm endoscopic periosteal elevator is used to carry the frontal subperiosteal dissection down the lateral orbital rim to the level of the infraorbital rim. If concurrent mid facelifting is planned, this dissection can be used to release the entire malar eminence.

6. Using the 30° endoscope for visualization, the frontal dissection is carried down to the supraorbital rim. The

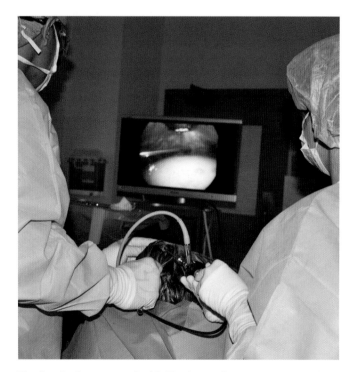

Fig. 5   Patient setup. Oral RAE tube used. Patient rotation of 90° away from anesthesia center allows for maximal access by surgeon and assistant with clear view of endoscope monitor.

endoscope is helpful for visualizing and avoiding transection of the supraorbital nerve (Fig. 7). The periosteum is incised along and parallel to the supraorbital rim using sharp and blunt dissectors. The dissection is carried around the supraorbital nerves if encountered.[5] Using a blunt curved dissector, the superior aspect of the cut periosteum is stretched 1 cm from the inferior edge. This maneuver helps prevent relapse of the surgical result.

7. The temporal incisions are then carried down to the temporoparietal fascia. If the superficial temporal vessels are encountered, they are ligated and moved from the dissection. After incising through the temporoparietal fascia, the dissection is carried bluntly down to the deep temporal fascia. A beaver-tail elevator is useful to bluntly open the superficial temporal space from 1 cm above the zygomatic arch to the superior temporal line. Dissection is carried anteriorly to the lateral orbital rim. It is important to only elevate inferiorly until a "soft stop" is encountered. This stop represents the confluence of deep and superficial temporal fascia, and further dissection places the frontal branch of the facial nerve at risk. The elevation of the superficial temporal space should also be carried posterior to the temporal incision until the entire space is open. This opening allows passive redraping of the temporal skin in a posterior-superior vector without the need to excise hair-bearing scalp.

8. An endoscope is inserted into the temporal incision to visualize the zygomaticotemporal bundle. This structure may be ligated if required to achieve passive elevation of the temporal skin.

9. A beaver-tail elevator is used to bluntly dissect through and release the temporoparietal fascia from the superior temporal line (Fig. 8). The elevator is inserted through the temporal incision and then used to sweep and release the fascia along the lateral orbital rim and superior temporal line. At this point, the forehead and temporal flaps should be contiguous and freely movable.

10. If desired for muscle hyperactivity, myotomies may be performed through the corrugator and procerus muscles using an electrocautery. The muscles are visualized by

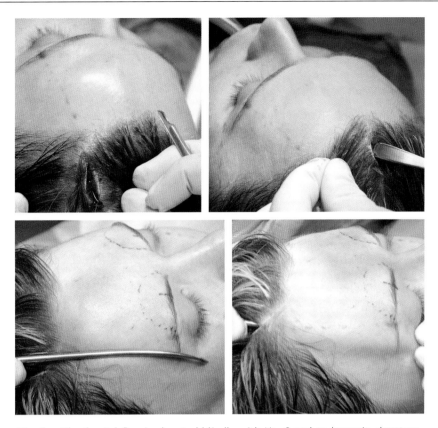

Fig. 6   The frontal flap is elevated blindly with No. 9 and endoscopic elevators.

retracting the cut periosteal edge superiorly, to expose the corrugators running diagonally just superficial to the periosteum. Similar myotomies may be carried through the lateral orbicularis oculi (crow's feet lines) and horizontally through the frontalis (forehead lines). Actual removal of the muscle bellies is generally not advised and may lead to contour deficiencies and unusual muscle contractions as a late postoperative complication.[5,6]

11. The forehead and temporal skin is assessed for passive elevation to the desired location. If there is still resistance to elevation, the site of resistance is determined and released; this is often due to inadequate release of periosteum along the supraorbital ridge and lateral orbital rim.

12. The temporal flap is secured in a posterior-superior vector using a 0-0 Nurulon or polydioxanone suture. The medial flap is secured through the temporoparietal fascia and secured with a hand tie to the deep temporal fascia. It is helpful to have an assistant "push" the temporal flap forcefully in the desired vector to allow maximal tightening. A second suture from inferior-medial temporoparietal fascia to superior-lateral deep temporal fascia is then placed to reinforce the lift (Fig. 9).

13. The frontal flap is then elevated and secured at the level of the paramedian incisions. The author prefers the resorbable Endotine devices to fixate the inferior flap periosteum to the underlying bone. Holes are drilled in the skull through the paramedian incisions to place the

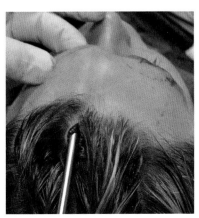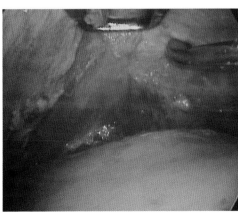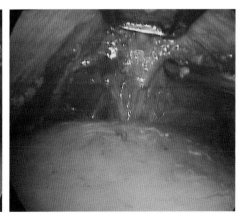

Fig. 7   The endoscope visualizes periosteal release, and the supraorbital nerve is visualized.

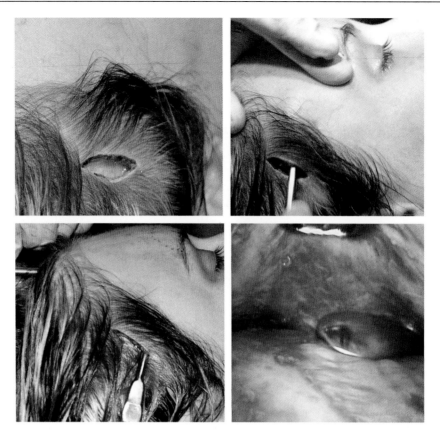

Fig. 8 The temporal dissection and conjoint tendon release as seen by endoscope inserted through parasagittal incision.

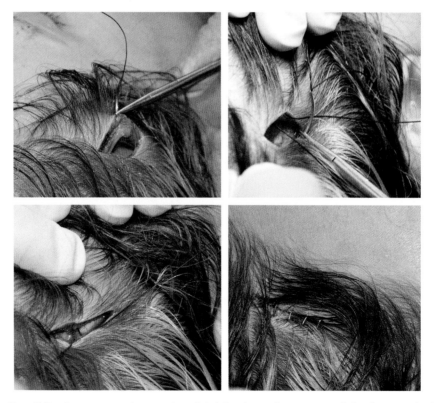

Fig. 9 Temporal dissection: 0-0 sutures secure temporal parietal fascia to deep temporal fascia posterior/superiorly. Closure with staples.

Endotine devices bilaterally. The inferior flap is then lifted off the bone and redraped superiorly with the help of an assistant. The Endotine prongs hold the periosteum in place (Fig. 10).

14. For brow height asymmetries, the surgeon will elevate the more dependent brow higher than its counterpart. After the forehead flap is secure, it is ideal to allow some time for any soft tissue creep to manifest itself. In a case with

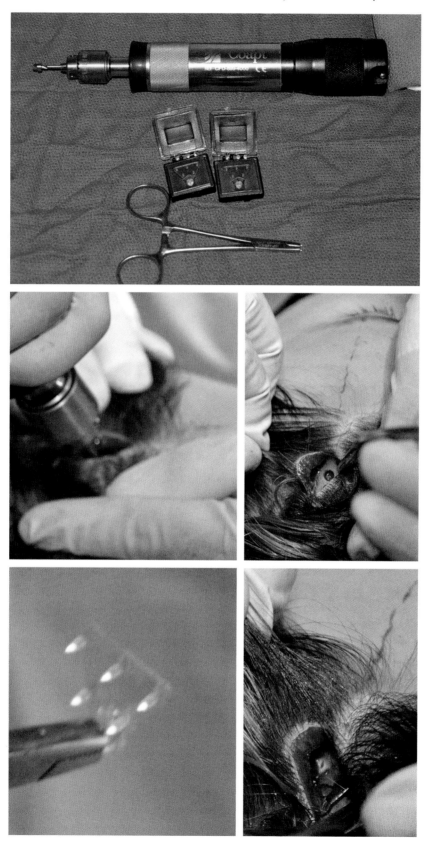

Fig. 10   Sequence for parasagittal Endotine placement.

multiple procedures, the brow height and forehead skin "tightness" are assessed at the end, and before finishing the case. If laxity of the brow and forehead has developed, the periosteum is detached from the Endotine device and it is again elevated and resecured under tension. The distance from the inferior brow at the level of maximum arch to the supraorbital rim is measured. In general, 4 to 6 mm of vertical relapse should be anticipated depending on the thickness and redundancy of the preoperative forehead. The brow is placed accordingly.

15. The incisions are then closed with staples. No dressings or drains are required. If a concurrent facelift is performed and a head wrap is placed, it is important to keep the wrap in a position as to elevate rather than depress the forehead skin. Bupivicaine 0.25% is infiltrated along the supraorbital rim and laterally to the level of the superior helix for patient comfort.

Postoperative technique
1. The patient is usually called on the night of surgery. It is not uncommon for patients to report severe tension headachelike discomfort. This pain typically resolves in 24 to 48 hours. Periorbital ecchymosis and edema are expected. A corticosteroid dose pack may be prescribed. The patient is allowed to gently rinse their hair on the second day, but is instructed not to put any forward and downward tension on the forehead flap. This instruction is recommended for 6 weeks.
2. Facial makeup is allowed by day 2, but often camouflage makeup is not effective until 5 to 7 days.
3. Staples are removed at 7 days.
4. Hair coloring may be performed at 1 month.
5. At 6 to 8 weeks, the result is considered stable. It is not uncommon that the Endotine devices are palpable out to 5 months (Fig. 11).

Technique key points
1. Specialized instruments are required to perform an endoscopic brow lift.
2. Preoperative marking is designed to elevate the maximal arch of the brow superiorly and slightly medially. The temporal flap is elevated posterior superiorly along a vector from ala to lateral canthus.
3. The endoscope is only used to visualize the dissection of the supraorbital and zygomaticotemporal bundles, and the periosteal release, and any modifications of the muscles of facial expression.
4. Recovery is typically uneventful with discomfort prominent for 24 to 48 hours.

Complications and controversies

Early complications
1. Hematoma
2. Loss of brow fixation/inadequate brow elevation
3. Weakness or paralysis of the frontal branch of the facial nerve
4. Loss of forehead/scalp sensation

Late complications
1. Dysesthesia, paresthesia, anesthesia of forehead and scalp
2. Relapse
3. Excessive medial brow elevation
4. Excessive interbrow distance
5. Frontal branch of facial nerve weakness/paralysis
6. Contour and muscle movement irregularities following myotomy

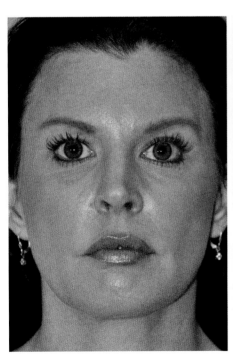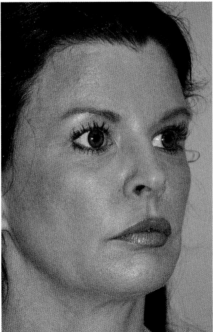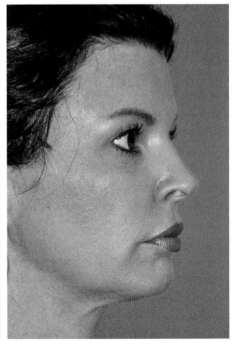

Fig. 11 Postoperative views at 1 year for endoscopic brow lift.

Hematoma

Hematomas should be evacuated when first noticed. Swelling and edema secondary to the hematoma increase the likihood of fixation failure.

Fixation failure

In the case of a recognizable failure of the fixation technique in the early (1–2 weeks) postoperative period, it is recommended to provide anesthesia and replace the fixation.

Facial nerve weakness/paralysis

Most facial nerve weaknesses resolve spontaneously. For symptomatic relief, botulinum toxin therapy to the working contralateral musculature is helpful. Function of the weakened side usually returns coincident with the end of the effect of botulinum toxin therapy.

Hypothesia/anesthesia of forehead and scalp

Hypothesia/anesthesia of forehead and scalp is usually self-limiting. Reassurance and forewarning are important. In cases that progress to problematic dysesthsia or paresthesia, a graduated corticosteroid pack is recommended. Low-dose amitryptyline 25 to 50 mg every night at bedtime is effective for reducing neurogenic discomfort and acting as a sleep aid.

The endoscopic brow lift is a relatively complication-free surgery. Major criticism is usually directed toward relapse/longevity of result, widening of the interbrow distance, and excessive medial brow elevation.

Avoiding relapse

1. Generous periosteal release with creation of 10-mm gap
2. Subperiosteal release of the lateral orbital rim to the level of the infraorbital rim
3. "Setting" the brow in position and then revisiting the lift at a later time in the surgery. If soft tissue creep has created laxity, the forehead flap is detached and replaced under tension.[1,6,7]

Avoiding excess interbrow distance and excessive medial brow elevation

1. The points of maximal brow arch are elevated in a superior and slightly medial direction; this tends to push the medial brow down relative to the arch and narrow the interbrow gap.
2. Avoid myotomies in the patient with a pre-existing wide or wide-normal interbrow distance. Corrugator myotomies coupled with temporal flap lateralization widens the interbrow distance. In cases with corrugator hyperactivity and wide interbrow distance, treatment with botulinum toxin is the preferred therapy over myotomy.

Complications key points

Most long-term complications of the endoscopic brow-lift procedure are related to inadequate periosteal release and fixation or utilization of improper vectors of pull and aggressive myotomy.

Other considerations

1. In the patient that would clearly benefit from a brow-lifting procedure but possesses a high hairline, a trichophytic approach is superior. In addition, the patient with a tall forehead creates an instrumentation difficulty as the endoscopic instruments may be of inadequate curve or length.
2. The coronal approach provides the best visualization if bony recontouring of the supraorbital and lateral orbital rim is desired.
3. In patients with Norwood male pattern hair loss grade 3 to 5, the 3 forehead incisions are abandoned in favor of 2 larger incisions at the height of the remaining temporal tuft. A horizontal 5-mm stab incision is made at the location that is desired for the Endotine device placement drill placement. In patients with Norwood 5 to 6 grade hair loss, a direct brow or midbrow lift approach may be preferable.
4. In men, upper blepharoplasty and endoscopic brow lift may easily be performed together. The patient is marked pre-operatively by the surgeon, while an assistant performs a simulated lift of the patient's brows.
5. In women. a simultaneous brow lift and upper blepharoplasty must be performed with caution. The patient is warned that the blepharoplasty will be more conservatively performed to avoid excess lagophthalmos and lid seal difficulties postoperatively. Ideally, the brow lift should be performed first, with the upper blepharoplasty to be performed after the resolution of edema in 2 to 4 months.
6. Lower blepharoplasty may be performed with the endoscopic brow lift without difficulty.

References

1. Core GB, Vasconez LO, Graham HD 3rd. Endoscopic browlift. Clin Plast Surg 1995;22(4):619–31.
2. Freund RM, Nolan WB 3rd. Correlation between brow lift outcomes and aesthetic ideals for eyebrow height and shape in females. Plast Reconstr Surg 1996;97(7):1343–8.
3. Gunter JP, Antrobus SD. Aesthetic analysis of the eyebrows. Plast Reconstr Surg 1997;99(7):1808–16.
4. Janis JE, Ghavami A, Lemmon JA, et al. Anatomy of the corrugator supercilii muscle: part I. Corrugator topography. Plast Reconstr Surg 2007;120(6):1647–53.
5. Janis JE, Ghavami A, Lemmon JA, et al. The anatomy of the corrugator supercilii muscle: part II. Supraorbital nerve branching patterns. Plast Reconstr Surg 2008;121(1):233–40.
6. Knoll BI, Attkiss KJ, Persing JA. The influence of forehead, brow, and periorbital aesthetics on perceived expression in the youthful face. Plast Reconstr Surg 2008;121(5):1793–802.
7. Matarasso A. Endoscopically assisted forehead-brow rhytidoplasty: theory and practice. Aesthetic Plast Surg 1995;19(2):141–7.

Management of Complications Associated with Upper Facial Rejuvenation

Angelo Cuzalina, MD, DDS [a],*, Manik Bedi, MD, DDS [b,1]

KEYWORDS

- Upper facial rejuvenation • Endoscopic browlift • Coronal browlift • Trichophytic browlift • Trichophylic browlift
- Browlift complications

KEY POINTS

- Upper facial rejuvenation is an important component of complete facial rejuvenation and has an overall low complication rate.
- Most complications of upper facial procedures are avoided with proper preoperative work-up, patient selection, diagnoses, and fundamental knowledge of relevant anatomy.
- With the advances in brow procedures, in particular the endoscopic forehead and brow lift, a more youthful appearance is achieved with avoiding an open procedure with unsightly scars.

Introduction

Patients who seek upper facial rejuvenation often present with complaints of excessive wrinkling, tired-appearing eyes, and excess eyelid skin. The goal of the cosmetic surgeon should be to restore the aesthetic balance and a youthful three-dimensional facial topography.[1] The cosmetic surgeon should take time to discuss the patient's goals and realistic outcomes including complications that may arise from the planned procedures. The conversation should include aging changes that occur in the upper facial region caused by

- Sun damage
- Gravity
- Bone resorption
- Decreased tissue elasticity
- Facial volume loss (deflation)
- Genetics

The facial aging process begins with surface and subsurface structural changes in multiple facial tissue layers, including skin, fat, muscle, and bone. These facial tissue layers age interdependently and contribute to the overall facial appearance.[1–4] The skin undergoes several changes including thinning, dryness, loss of elasticity, reduction in collagen, and increased likeliness to wrinkle or sag.[4] The collagen loss is a key factor and decreases the skin's ability to retain elasticity

(elastin) and moisture (hyaluronic acid). The aging face has redistribution, accumulation, and atrophy of fat that leads to an overall facial volume loss.[5] There is also loss of craniofacial bone with age and without this structural support there are perceptible changes in the overlying layers.[3,4]

Upper facial rejuvenation procedures rank at the top of facial cosmetics with more than 206,000 blepharoplasties performed in 2014 (number two of all facial cosmetic surgical procedures) and 42,000 forehead lifts in 2014 (number five of all facial cosmetic surgical procedures). The top minimally invasive cosmetic procedures for 2014 were botulinum toxin type A (6.7 million) and soft tissue fillers (2.3 million). A thorough preoperative evaluation, knowledge of pertinent anatomy, and meticulous surgical planning allow cosmetic surgeons to prevent and understand the management of complications (Fig. 1).

Preoperative evaluation

Preoperative risk assessment should take into account the patient's overall health status (American Society of Anesthesiologists [ASA] physical status); fortunately most patient's presenting for facial cosmetic surgery are healthy (ASA I) or have a mild, controlled systemic disease (ASA II). Preexisting cardiovascular disease, particularly systemic hypertension, should be well controlled because it may predispose the patient to hematoma formation. Facial cosmetic surgical procedures carry a low (<1%) risk of major cardiac complications, such as cardiac death or nonfatal myocardial infarction.[6] Preoperative 12-lead electrocardiogram and routine preoperative laboratory testing should be performed as indicated. Pulmonary status of patients with chronic obstructive pulmonary disease should be evaluated and optimized to decrease the chance of postoperative pulmonary complications. In particular, cigarette smoking is associated with a 12- to 20-fold increase in flap slough and excessive

Disclosure Statement: The authors have nothing to disclose.
[a] Private Practice, Tulsa Surgical Arts, 7322 East 91st Street, Tulsa, OK 74133, USA
[b] Private Practice, 6153 Fort King Road, Zephyrhills, FL 33542, USA
* Corresponding author.
E-mail address: angelo@tulsasurgicalarts.com
[1] Present address: 6153 Fort King Road, Zephyrhills, FL 33542.

Atlas Oral Maxillofacial Surg Clin N Am 24 (2016) 175-180
1061-3315/16/$ - see front matter © 2016 Elsevier Inc. All rights reserved.
http://dx.doi.org/10.1016/j.cxom.2016.05.001

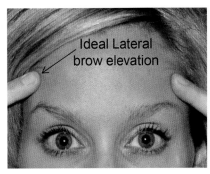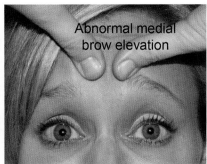

Fig. 1 Photographs depict why some browlift patients have a bizarre look from a potential complication of overelevation of the medial brow. Lateral brow elevation looks attractive on most females but medial brow elevation greater than the lateral brow third creates an odd look for male or female browlift patients.

coughing postoperatively caused by abnormal airway reactivity can increase the risk of postoperative bleeding.[7,8] Patients should be instructed to discontinue smoking and nicotine products for a minimum 3 weeks before and after surgery. Patients with diabetes mellitus and rheumatologic disease should be medically optimized before surgery because they are prone to bruising, infection, and delayed healing (Fig. 2). A personal or family history of blood dyscrasias should be noted. The use of the following should be stopped at least 2 weeks before surgery to avoid the risk of excessive bleeding:

- Nonsteroidal anti-inflammatory drugs
- Aspirin
- Fish oil
- Herbal supplements, such as ginkgo, *Echinacea*, and St. John's wort
- Certain vitamins (eg, vitamin E)

Patients with obesity and history of a difficult airway should be evaluated for sleep-disordered breathing. Obstructive sleep apnea is screened for using a simple STOP-BANG questionnaire.[9]

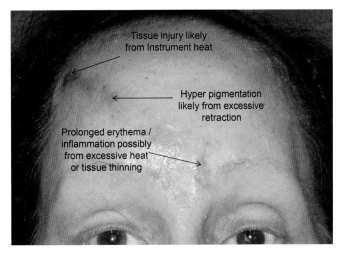

Fig. 2 Photograph demonstrating several complications in a female patient. Most seem caused by excess trauma from heat and improper retraction. Extremely thin patients or patients who smoke are at a higher risk for these types of complications because their margin for error is narrowed. The layers of the brow can be very thin particularly after superficial muscle resection. Gentle tissue manipulation is critical to avoid these types of issues.

Complications in browlift

Procedures to lift the ptotic brow were initially described by Hunt[10] in 1926 and later in 1930, Passot discussed the direct browlift with an excision of an ellipse of tissue above the brow.[11] The endoscopic brow lifting was first introduced in 1991 by Keller.[12] The overall complication rate for any forehead procedure is low. De Cordier and coworkers[13] retrospectively reviewed 393 patients who underwent endoscopic forehead lift from 1994 to 2000. The review reported alopecia in one occurrence (0.3%), transient scalp numbness in most patients, 2% with prolonged dysesthesia, and seven patients (2.3%) with a temporary frontal nerve weakness. Forehead hematoma requiring in-office drainage occurred in 3.5% of patients. Seven percent of their patients experienced lagophthalmos, 8% with upper eyelid asymmetry, and 3% with brow malposition. There was also one patient who had wound dehiscence and one who had a suture abscess.

Brow malposition

For successful rejuvenation the surgeon must have a fundamental knowledge of forehead anatomy. In the forehead, the layers are.[14]

- Skin
- Subcutaneous tissue
- Muscle
- Fibrous galea
- Loose areolar tissue
- Pericranium

The superficial musculoaponeurotic system in the lower two-thirds of the face continues as the superficial temporoparietal fascia over the zygoma and then merges with the fibrous galea in the forehead. The temporal line is formed by the convergence of the deep and superficial layers of the deep temporal fascia. The deep temporal fascia is thicker and has a white glistening appearance. Inferior to the zygomatic arch, the deep temporal fascia splits into two layers called the intermediate temporal and deep temporal fasciae. Another important landmark in brow lifting procedures is the adherent arcus marginalis along the supraorbital rim, this is where the periosteum of the frontal bone fuses with the galea. Release of these dense fibrous attachments in forehead rejuvenation is important to produce the desired elevation and stabilization of the brow. Preoperative evaluation of the patient with photographic documentation noting asymmetries helps minimize the risk of patient dissatisfaction. Careful patient selection, release of arcus marginalis, and symmetric suspension should decrease the risk of poor patient satisfaction.

Malposition of the brow may occur with any approach to forehead rejuvenation.[15] Too much resection of skin in any open approach or excessive suspension with any procedure may results in possible lagophthalmos and brow malposition (Fig. 3). The risk is increased when simultaneously blepharoplasty is performed. To avoid excessive skin resection during the blepharoplasty the forehead lift should be completed before the eyelid surgery. When lagophthalmos is limited to less than 2 mm there is a decreased risk of dry eye syndrome.[16] If a patient develops symptoms of irritation or dryness this should be treated with lubricating eye drops and ointments. In one study of 600 patients who underwent combined upper blepharoplasty and open coronal browlift there was no dry eye syndrome, blindness, or globe exposure, and there were only two cases of brow asymmetry.[17] In a retrospective study comparing 140 (121 coronal and 19 endoscopic) patients who had either the endoscopic-assisted approach or the open approach there was no significant difference in brow elevation with either approach alone or in combination with blepharoplasty at the 1-year evaluation.[18]

When there is overelevation of the brow, consideration should be made to perform release of the suspension. When there is underelevation of the brow this likely caused by inadequate release, fixation, or suspension. This is treated with revision surgery and ensuring proper release, suspension, or skin excision. Overresection of the depressor supercilli can lead to medial overelevation and a "surprised" appearance. This is avoided by recognition of the anatomy intraoperative. Minor asymmetries are improved with strategic placement of neurotoxins.

Nerve damage

Sensory disturbances should be discussed with patient preoperatively. Peri-incisional anesthesia is expected and is usually temporary. The supraorbital and supratrochlear nerves should be preserved to minimize forehead hypothesia medially up to the vertex. To help locate these important structures a preoperative mark should be made along a vertical line through the brow parallel to the medial limbus (iris) while the patient faces forward. The supraorbital vessels and nerves typically lie within 1 mm of this mark at the orbital rim 98% of the time. This was reproduced with a study using a needle through a skin mark and visualization of the neurovascular position endoscopically. The supratrochlear nerve exits from around the orbital rim approximately 1 cm medial to the exit of the supraorbital nerve.[19] Direct injury to the nerves is an uncommon occurrence but traction injury (neuropraxia) can occur because of suspension. When neuropraxia injury occurs it may take up to 12 months to completely resolve. In the temporal region the dissection plane is superficial to the superficial layer of the deep temporal fascia and damage to the

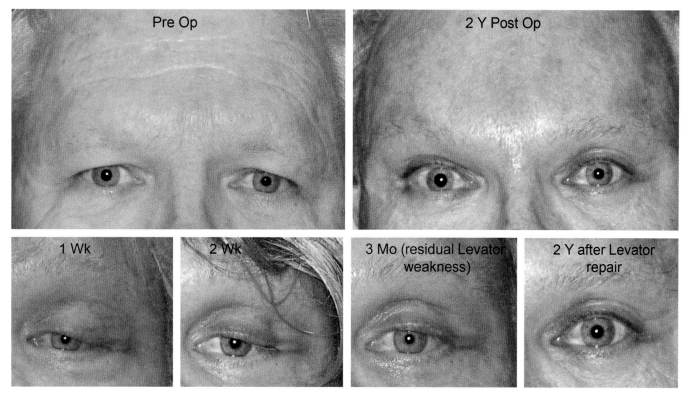

Fig. 3 A 67-year-old transgender patient shown before and 2 years following a coronal browlift, blepharoplasties, and frontal bossing bone reduction. The lower set of photographs show a complication that occurred resulting from profound edema around the left eye. Despite slow improvement over a period of 3 to 6 months, complete resolution never resolved. The trauma likely damaged the levator muscle and aponeurosis from the profound swelling and a classic "A frame" deformity can be seen at 3 months postoperative. An anterior levator repair was performed at 9 months to correct the problem.

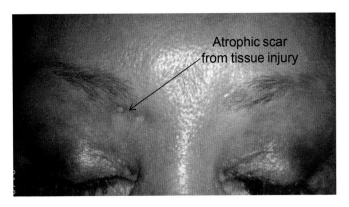

Fig. 4 The atrophic scar show is from various causes during a browlift. The most common reason for this complication is excessive thinning of tissue during corrugator muscle resection. Other potential reasons are an inadvertent perforation with any instrument or excess heat from electrocautery. The heat injuries tend to take the longest to heal and care must be always taken to ensure proper electrocautery settings and proper suction placement to remove excess heat.

zygomaticotemporal and auricotemporal nerves (second division of trigeminal) should be minimal.

The facial nerve and its branches must be known to avoid injury because this results in paralysis and asymmetry of the forehead. In particular, the temporal (frontal) branch is at risk for injury in the temporal lateral dissection. In a 1979 article by Al-Kayat and Bramley[20] the location of the facial nerve's main trunk was described and found that it runs no nearer than 1.5 cm below the inferior margin of the bony external auditory meatus and that the most posterior temporal branch of the nerve crosses the zygomatic arch anterior to the bony external auditory meatus at a minimum distance of 0.8 cm and mean of 2.0 cm. A more recent high-resolution MRI study of live subjects measured a minimum distance of 1.7 cm and mean of 2.1 cm.[21] Another anatomic study of interest discussed the facial nerve's path in three dimensions. The study showed that the temporal branch lies in the loose areolar connective tissue layer between the superficial and deep temporal fascia as it crosses the zygomatic arch; it enters the superficial temporal fascia from its undersurface in a consistent region 1.5 cm to 3.0 cm above the zygomatic arch and 0.9 cm to 1.4 cm posterior to the lateral orbital rim.[22]

The zone of fixation that begins at the lateral corner of the superior orbital rim must be released and during this dissection the temporal branch of the facial nerve can be damaged. In this area the lateral oribuclaris oculi is exposed and precise release where all the fascial layers come together prevents nerve injury. Another structure that is of importance in this lateral corner is the sentinel vein, which is situated approximately 1 cm lateral to the zygomaticofrontal suture line.

Scars

Scarring is of concern with open browlift procedures and typically results from improper incision design and closure. The unsightly scar may be minimized in open approaches by making an irregular incision with an extreme bevel from posterior to anterior beginning 4 to 5 mm posterior to the hairline at an area where the follicular density becomes consistent. The extreme bevel of the incision preserves the hair follicles on the superior flap allowing hair growth through and anterior to the scar postoperatively.[23] Scarring and thinning of tissue caused by overzealous resection of brow elevators are best managed by dermabrasion or fillers (Fig. 4).

Alopecia

Alopecia can also result from improper incision design and closure, including inappropriate wound tension, and excessive use of electrocautery. Peri-incisional alopecia can appear as a widened scar; when the scar is visible by the endoscopic approach, the scar can be excised at a later date. Alopecia around endoscopic scars can make them more obvious and scar revision can be performed to improve the scars by excision of the widened scars and closed reapproximation of the hair-bearing scalp. As an alternative, follicular unit hair transplants can be placed in the scar.

Acute tellogen effluvium is a rare but known cause of hair loss after brow procedures (Fig. 5). The features include diffuse shedding sometimes with accentuated hair thinning, a normal-appearing scalp, and a markedly positive pull test. The hair pull test is done by grasping approximately 40 to 60 hairs between the thumb and index finger and applying steady traction (slightly stretching the scalp) as you slide your fingers along the length of the hair. Generally, only a few hairs in the

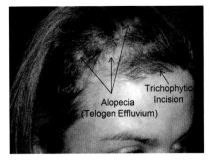
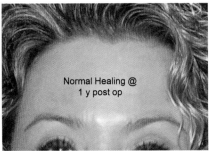

Fig. 5 The patient shown had a classic trichophytic browlift without any early problems. However, she developed severe alopecia (hair loss) approximately 2 months following surgery known as telogen effluvium. The patient had complete healing with time. The only treatment was early low-dose steroid injections and minor topical hair growth medication usage. Fortunately, most cases resolve spontaneously.

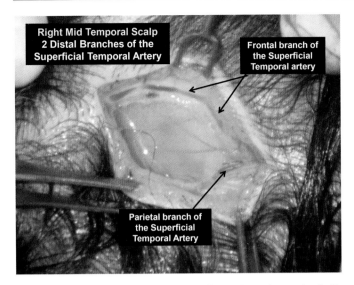

Fig. 6 The right temporal scalp is shown just above the helix of the ear in an incision location for a lateral endoscopic port incision or a temporal lift. Two branches of the superficial temporary artery are shown that are seen in the upper temporoparietal fascia. They are one of many sources for hematoma or at minimum a nuisance to a clean operating field.

telogen (resting) phase can be plucked in this fashion. Less than 10% is considered normal, whereas greater than this is considered indicative of a pathologic process.[24] Fortunately, tellogen effluvium is a self-resolving condition and regrowth is noted in 3 to 6 months, but cosmetically significant regrowth can take 12 to 18 months.

Bleeding

Excessive bleeding may occur with any approach and may be arterial, venous, or from skin edges (Fig. 6). Preoperative evaluation to note blood dyscrasias and patient education on avoidance of agents that cause bleeding prevent most issues. Injection with a hemostatic agent, ensuring intraoperative hemostasis, and avoidance of injury to the superficial temporal or zygomaticotemporal arteries, supraorbital or supratrochlear vascular bundles, and sentinel vein decreases postoperative hematomas. If there is slow postoperative bleeding it may be controlled with pressure alone, although hematomas require evacuation, exploration, and control of bleeding.

Summary

Cosmetic procedures of the upper third of the face is frequently an essential component for complete facial rejuvenation. Upper facial rejuvenation has had many advances over the years from the traditional coronal lift and direct browlift and to the trichophylic and trichophytic modifications. Most recently in the past two decades the endoscopic approach has been incorporated as a popular means to provide long-lasting results with low complications. Regardless of the approach, a more youthful appearance is achieved and complications can be minimized by a thorough preoperative history and physical examination, proper patient selection and diagnoses, meticulous surgical technique, appropriate suspension, and a tension-free wound closure.

References

1. Murphy MR, Johnson CM Jr, Azizzadeh B. The aging face consultation. In: Master techniques in facial rejuvenation. Philadelphia: Saunders Elsevier; 2007. p. 1–16.
2. Coleman SR, Grover R. The anatomy of the aging face: volume loss and changes in 3-dimensional topography. Aesthet Surg J 2006; 26(Suppl 1):S4–9.
3. Zimbler MS, Kokoska MS, Thomas JR. Anatomy and pathophysiology of facial aging. Facial Plast Surg Clin North Am 2001;9:179–87.
4. Vleggaar D, Fitzgerald R. Dermatological implications of skeletal aging: a focus on supraperiosteal volumization for perioral rejuvenation. J Drugs Dermatol 2008;7:209–20.
5. Donofrio LM. Fat distribution: a morphologic study of the aging face. Dermatol Surg 2000;26:1107–12.
6. Fleisher LA, Beckman JA, Brown KA, et al. ACC/AHA 2007 guidelines on perioperative cardiovascular evaluation and care for noncardiac surgery: a report of the American College of Cardiology/American Heart Association Task Force on Practice Guidelines (Writing Committee to Revise the 2002 Guidelines on Perioperative Cardiovascular Evaluation for Noncardiac Surgery) developed in collaboration with the American Society of Echocardiography, American Society of Nuclear Cardiology, Heart Rhythm Society, Society of Cardiovascular Anesthesiologists, Society for Cardiovascular Angiography and Interventions, Society for Vascular Medicine and Biology, and Society for Vascular Surgery. J Am Coll Cardiol 2007;50:e159–241.
7. Prendiville S, Weiser S. Management of anesthesia and facility in facelift surgery. Facial Plast Surg Clin North Am 2009;17:531–8.
8. Clevens RA. Avoiding patient dissatisfaction and complications in facelift surgery. Facial Plast Surg Clin North Am 2009;17:515–30.
9. Chung F, Yegneswaran B, Liao P, et al. STOP questionnaire: a tool to screen patients for obstructive sleep apnea. Anesthesiology 2008;108:812–21.
10. Hunt HL. Plastic surgery of the head, face and neck. Philadelphia: Lea and Febinger; 1926.
11. Passot R. Chirurgie esthetique pure: techniques et results. Paris (France): Gaston Doin et Cie; 1930.
12. Keller GS. Endolaser excision of glabellar frown lines and forehead rhytids. Paper Presented at a Meeting of the American Academy of Facial Plastic and Reconstructive Surgery. Los Angeles, February 1, 1992.
13. De Cordier BC, de la Torre JI, Al-Hakeem MS, et al. Endoscopic forehead lift: review of technique, cases, and complications. Plast Reconstr Surg 2002;110(6):1558–68.
14. O'Brien JX, Ashton MW, Rozen WM, et al. New perspectives on the surgical anatomy and nomenclature of the temporal region: literature review and dissection study. Plast Reconstr Surg 2013;131(3): 510–22.
15. Guyurn B. Endoscopic forehead rejuvenation: I. Limitations, flaws, and rewards. Plast Reconstr Surg 2006;117(4):1121–33.
16. Terella AM, Wang TD, Kim MM. Complications in periorbital surgery. Facial Plast Surg 2013;29(1):64–70.
17. Friedland JA, Jacobsen WM, TerKonda S. Safety and efficacy of combined upper blepharoplasties and open coronal browlift: a consecutive series of 600 patients. Aesthetic Plast Surg 1996;20(6): 453–62.
18. Dayan SH, Perkins SW, Vartanian AJ, et al. The forehead lift: endoscopic versus coronal approaches. Aesthetic Plast Surg 2001; 25(1):35–9.
19. Cuzalina A, Holmes D. A simple and reliable landmark for identification of the supraorbital nerve in surgery of the forehead: an in vivo anatomical study. J Oral Maxillofac Surg 2005;63:25–7.
20. Al-Kayat A, Bramley P. A modified pre-auricular approach to the temporomandibular joint and malar arch. Br J Oral Surg 1979;17: 91–103.
21. Miloro M, Redlinger S, Pennington DM, et al. In situ location of the temporal branch of the facial nerve. J Oral Maxillofac Surg 2007; 65(12):2466–9.

22. Agarwal CA, Mendenhall SD, Foreman KB, et al. The course of the frontal branch of the facial nerve in relation to fascial planes: an anatomic study. Plast Reconstr Surg 2010;125(2):532–7.

23. Owsley TG. Subcutaneous trichophytic forehead browlift: the case for an "open" approach. J Oral Maxillofac Surg 2006;64(7):1133–6.

24. Piérard GE, Piérard-Franchimont C, Marks R, et alfor the EEMCO group (European Expert Group on Efficacy Measurement of Cosmetics and Other Topical Products). EEMCO guidance for the assessment of hair shedding and alopecia. Skin Pharmacol Physiol 2004;17(2):98–110.

Moving?

Make sure your subscription moves with you!

To notify us of your new address, find your **Clinics Account Number** (located on your mailing label above your name), and contact customer service at:

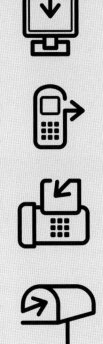

Email: journalscustomerservice-usa@elsevier.com

800-654-2452 (subscribers in the U.S. & Canada)
314-447-8871 (subscribers outside of the U.S. & Canada)

Fax number: 314-447-8029

Elsevier Health Sciences Division
Subscription Customer Service
3251 Riverport Lane
Maryland Heights, MO 63043

*To ensure uninterrupted delivery of your subscription, please notify us at least 4 weeks in advance of move.